PRAISE FOR

MENTAL FITNESS

"In this latest book *Mental Fitness,* Shawn Talbott draws from scientific, anecdotal and personal information to highlight the dramatic challenges to our mental wellness, and shows practical ways how to prevent and to effectively deal with the continuous rise in a wide range of physical and mental diseases we are currently experiencing. An important read for anybody who is sick of covering up the underlying problems with medications and explore non-pharmaceutical solutions."

–**Emeran A. Mayer,** MD, Distinguished Professor at UCLA
and author of *The Mind Gut Connection* and *The Gut-Immune Connection*

❧

"Dr. Shawn Talbott is an expert in the scientific fields of functional nutrition, functional medicine as well as in functional food science. By using different approaches including functional medicine he is trying to get to the root cause of disease and trying to improve both mental and physical performance."

–**Dr. Danik Martirosyan,** PhD, Editor-in-Chief, FFHD.
President, Functional Food Center, Functional Food Institute

❧

"Dr. Shawn Talbott is one of the top thinkers of our time concerning the intersection between nutrition, physical and mental performance and mental health.

Mental Fitness is the culmination of decades of Shawn's cutting edge research and work, integrating the latest science in an easy-to-understand manner."

–**Kerry Hughes,** Ethnobotanist, Herbalist and Author

"As a fitness professional with 30 years of experience, I couldn't be more elated with the timing of Dr. Shawn Talbott's book, *Mental Fitness*. This is the secret sauce in creating long term, sustainable and holistic wellness. Shawn not only has a way of making complicated scientific information digestible, he also is a perfect role model of how to apply what he teaches. This book will be a resource I will turn to frequently for myself and my clients."

–**Kat Morrill,** CPT, CHC, CGF,
Master Fitness Educator and Global Fitness Consultant

MENTAL FITNESS

Maximizing
Mood, Motivation, & Mental Wellness
by Optimizing the Brain-Body-Biome

SHAWN M. TALBOTT
PHD, CNS, LDN, FACSM, FACN

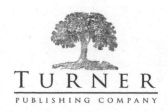

TURNER
PUBLISHING COMPANY

Turner Publishing Company
Nashville, TN
www.turnerpublishing.com

ISBNs: 9781684426768 (paperback)
        9781684426775 (hardback)
        9781684426782 (ebook)

Library of Congress Control Number: 2021021856

Cover design by Nicolette Donohoe and Grace Cavalier
Interior design by Gary A. Rosenberg

Printed in the United States of America
17 18 19 20 10 9 8 7 6 5 4 3 2

CONTENTS

PREFACE

MENTAL FITNESS

At no time in human history have we ever been so "advanced" techno-logically and yet so miserable psychologically.

It's no exaggeration to describe stress, depression, anxiety, and burn-out as epidemics—literally the "black plague" of our modern times.

We'll get into the reasons we feel so terrible soon enough in the chapters to come. But how you feel is not just in your head; it's also in your gut, your heart, your immune system, and in many other places inside and outside your actual brain.

I've been researching, speaking, and writing about the mental fitness topics covered in this book for more than twenty years, and I've written a dozen previous books on related topics.

I started writing this particular volume in early 2019 as a way to bring together some of the most exciting scientific breakthroughs around the "gut-heart-brain axis" linking psychology, neurology, biochemistry, physi-ology, and microbiology into the emerging field of nutritional psychology (which is what the area of my expertise is now commonly called). At the start of 2019, I really didn't think that our collective mental wellness problems could get much worse.

Boy, was I wrong!

National surveys showed that happiness and life-satisfaction levels were at all-time lows, while depression, suicide, drug addiction, and use of prescription antidepressants and pain-killing opioids were at all-time highs.

And then COVID-19 hit.

In the first weeks of 2020, we began to see the emergence of COVID-19 and its subsequent spread around the globe devastating health systems, economies, and individuals—both physically and mentally.

At the time of this writing, more than 100 million COVID-19 cases with now over 3 million deaths have been recorded worldwide—with more than 32 million cases and 500,000 deaths in the United States alone.

The COVID-19 pandemic resulted in more than half the world's population being placed under different levels of quarantines and lockdowns to stem the spread of the virus. These restrictions are expected to significantly influence the physical and psychological well-being of everyone affected. Research studies are already showing a clear and consistent increase in mental health issues around the globe, particularly among adolescents and young adults.

Some of the reasons underlying the increase in mental health problems are biological, some are psychological, and some are financial, but they all coalesce toward numerous predictions of a looming mental health crisis that was already bad and is only expected to get worse in a post-COVID world.

I hope you agree with me that there is no physical health without mental health. They are two sides of the same coin, and they are vital for each other and for our ability to reach our peak potential in this one life we have to live.

We will cover many of these topics in *Mental Fitness*, and we'll consider how research-supported natural approaches can improve how we feel mentally and perform physically in every aspect of our daily lives.

Thanks for joining me.

Shawn Talbott
Salt Lake City, Utah, USA
February 24, 2021

INTRODUCTION

WHAT IS MENTAL FITNESS?

It might surprise you to realize that the biggest health problems today are not physical ailments such as heart disease, cancer, diabetes, and Alzheimer's disease but rather are mental conditions such as depression, anxiety, chronic fatigue, sleep deprivation, and everyday stress. In many ways—including biochemically, physiologically, and behaviorally—"mental wellness" is the overarching umbrella that determines our overall physical health, and "mental fitness" can be thought of as the optimized state of mental wellness.

For example, when we're stressed, we're more likely to crave junk food and store belly fat, but when we're resilient, we don't succumb to stress-eating and we make better dietary choices. When we're tired, we're less likely to exercise or meditate, but when we have good sleep quality and metabolism, we have abundant energy levels that can fuel our lifestyle. When we're depressed, we're less likely to take care of ourselves or interact positively with others, but when we have a good mood, we're more likely to love ourselves and apply that love to others.

Each of these aspects of mental wellness, and ultimately mental fitness, drives a specific change in behavior that leads to a negative or positive impact on physical health.

Imagine if your "default state" was inclined toward mental fitness.

Imagine having naturally high levels of energy so you feel like being physically active on a daily basis.

Imagine being resilient in the face of whatever stressors you encounter on a daily basis so that rather than stepping away from stressful events, you can step into them and take care of business.

Imagine having a naturally positive outlook on life that infects others with positivity rather than a negative and pessimistic view of the world and your place in it.

This book will help you understand how optimizing your mental fitness can not only help you feel better (both quickly and long-term) but also how those changes can improve your physical health—including how you look and perform on every level.

According to the World Health Organization, *mental health* is defined as "a state of well-being in which every individual

➤ realizes his or her own potential,

➤ can cope with the normal stresses of life,

➤ can work productively and fruitfully,

➤ and is able to make a contribution to his or her community."

Mental wellness exists on a continuum across

➤ depression, anxiety, and burnout on the low end ("struggling"),

➤ to daily stress, nightly restlessness, and feeling "blah" ("typical"),

➤ to abundant energy, sharpness, creativity, vigor, and thriving on the high end of mental fitness ("optimized").

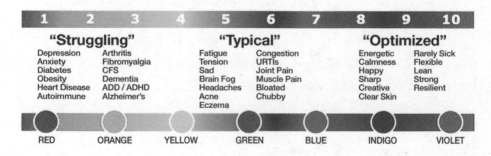

MENTAL FITNESS CONTINUUM

The Problem

The World Health Organization (WHO) has identified stress and depression as global epidemics and the leading causes of disability worldwide. In North America alone, hundreds of millions of people spend hundreds of billions of dollars every year on "feel different" remedies such as antidepressant and antianxiety drugs, opioid painkillers, drugs for ADHD, drugs for sleep, and an unending array of energy drinks and junk food that we self-medicate with in response to being tired, stressed, and depressed.

Unfortunately, while many of these approaches will change how we feel, none of them will help us feel better. These synthetic approaches generally take us from feeling bad in one way to feeling bad in a different way. They utterly fail to help us feel the way we want to feel—good.

The Disconnect

In the last fifty years, health-care spending on a per-person basis in the United States has increased by more than 2,000 percent, but I would wager that we're less healthy in many ways today than we were five decades ago. According to the WHO, the United States has the most expensive health-care system in the world (by far), yet the overall health and well-being of its citizens ranks near the bottom of industrialized countries (seventy-second overall).

The modern disease-care model gobbles up more than 20 percent of the entire American economy—and the largest portion of those expenditures are for the categories of prescription drugs targeting "physical pain" and "psychological pain." The "physical pain" drugs include a wide range of anti-inflammatory and analgesic drugs, including opioids. The "psychological pain" drugs encompass an even wider range of antidepressants, tranquilizers, and sleep aids. Not quite as large, but growing more rapidly, are costs associated with drugs for gut problems such as irritable bowel syndrome (IBS) and Crohn's disease; drugs for brain problems such as attention deficit hyperactivity disorder (ADHD), autism spectrum disorders, and Alzheimer's disease; and drugs for heart problems such as cardiovascular disease and hypertension.

These broad categories of modern afflictions—physical imbalances in the gut, brain, and body leading to emotional imbalances in how we feel mentally, physically, and spiritually—are exploding to epidemic levels with never-before-seen increases in the incidence of depression, anxiety, burnout, ADHD, autism, insomnia, Alzheimer's, chronic fatigue syndrome, fibromyalgia, and post-traumatic stress disorder (PTSD).

The Current "Solutions" Have Failed

It seems that our massive health-care expenditures, especially on prescription drugs, are badly missing the mark in helping improve our physical health or our mental wellness. Think for just a minute about whether someone you know, including yourself, suffers from one of the more common "brain" symptoms: stress, trouble focusing (or being easily distracted), brain fog, daytime fatigue, nighttime restlessness, or trouble falling asleep. If you fall into this category of "tired, stressed, and depressed," then you're in good company.

➤ More than sixty million Americans have depression and/or anxiety.

➤ One in five Americans takes a mood-altering drug, including antidepressants, antianxiety drugs, sleep drugs, and ADHD drugs.

➤ Alzheimer's disease will affect as much as 50 percent of our population over the age of eighty-five (the fastest-growing segment).

➤ More than 10 percent of kids are affected by ADHD, with many drugged on methylphenidate (Ritalin) and related drugs that are chemically similar to methamphetamines (a.k.a. "meth").

➤ Autism spectrum disorders, including Asperger's, rates have skyrocketed by more than ten times in the last five to ten years (now reaching about 1 in 166 kids).

Sources of stress in our modern 24-7 always-on world are endless, including psychological, physical, cellular, environmental, socioeconomic, and social (as well as the growing epidemic of loneliness that is closely related to mental wellness—more on that later).

While my own research has focused for nearly two decades on the links between nutrition, biochemistry, and psychology—considering how and why nutrients make us feel a certain way—none of us are immune to struggles with mental wellness. In the past, members of my own family, including myself, have battled feelings of stress, depression, and addiction, but now we're at an exciting time in history where we can finally use traditional natural options to address many of today's modern mental wellness challenges.

The last few years have seen fundamental changes in our scientific understanding of mental wellness. This leads us in new directions for improving mental wellness, enhancing mental fitness, and optimizing mental performance. *Mental Fitness* focuses on these breakthroughs in our understanding of ancient/traditional medicine and natural lifestyle factors such as nutrition/supplements, exercise/movement, sleep/stress, and many others to provide us with a wide array of scientifically validated tools that can dramatically improve how we feel and perform in every aspect of our lives.

A New Solution—Our Three Brains

The "first" brain in your head is networked with both the gut (our "second" brain) and with the heart (our "third" brain). Each of our three brains sends and receives a wide range of signals to and from each other, and each has its own strengths and weaknesses.

It is the coordinated action of our three brains—and the interplay among them—that ultimately determines our overall mental wellness.

The thinking brain in our head certainly perceives our emotions and determines our behaviors. But what our first brain perceives is dependent on what it receives in terms of the signals coming from other parts of the body, such as the gut and the heart (our two other brains). The brain in the head receives these signals and integrates them into a decision, emotion, or explanation of the world around us and helps determine where we fall on the mental wellness continuum and our overall level of mental fitness.

Brain	Function	Strength
Head (first) = "Mind"	Thinking brain (logic/logos)	Logical
Gut (second) = "Body"	Sensing brain (emotion/pathos)	Intuitive
Heart (third) = "Spirit"	Feeling brain (trust/ethos)	Empathetic

The "sensing" brain in our gut and the "feeling" brain in our heart are the primary generators of signals to our "thinking" brain in our head. We need to have coherence (versus incoherence) and resonance (versus dissonance) across our three brains for optimal mental fitness. It's a partnership among the brains, a collaboration, and we can optimize those signals that our first brain receives from the gut and heart to help move us up the mental wellness continuum.

Our three brains "talk" to each other through a complex network of nerves, cells, and biochemicals. This network—referred to as the gut-heart-brain axis—includes nearly one hundred trillion bacteria that live in our gastrointestinal system (our "microbiome") and the cloud of electrical and magnetic signals generated by our heart. Coordination between these helpful bacteria and coherent heart signals are instrumental in modulating the function of our immune system, optimizing the body's inflammatory response, and supporting many other aspects of our mental wellness and physical health.

Mental Fitness

The term *vigor* is one way to describe mental fitness. In research studies of interventions to help people feel better, "vigor" is defined as "a sustained

3-tiered mood state characterized by physical energy, mental acuity, and emotional well-being." In psychology research, "vigor" is also the opposite state from "burnout."

I've been studying vigor for at least the last twenty years, and in those two decades our understanding of what improves and what degrades vigor has undergone some meaningful changes. We used to think that vigor was "just" related to the brain and various influences of stress hormones such as cortisol. Eventually, science advanced enough to inform us that the microbiome (the collection of trillions of gut bacteria) creates up to 90 percent of the body's neurotransmitters such as serotonin and dopamine and has a dramatic influence on mood, motivation, and resilience. Even more recent are the scientific and medical observations that the heart, through electromagnetic signals sent to the brain, plays an equally influential role in determining our mental well-being.

My usage of the term *diet* is intended to encompass not just the diet of the food we eat but also our "diet" of physical activity that we "feed" to our body and our "diet" of thoughts that we "feed" to our brain. The word *diet* is most properly defined simply as "habitual exposure," so whatever we expose ourselves to on a regular basis—including foods, supplements, exercise, thoughts, experiences, people, and more—becomes the "diet" nourishing our three brains (and the axis among them) and determining our level of mental fitness.

I've written several best-selling books about the concept of vigor, including how to use natural approaches to bolster vigor in the face of modern stressors. This book and the "mental fitness" terminology are my attempt to expand on those ideas and broaden the well-being benefits by bringing together the latest scientific understandings about how our three brains (head/gut/heart) and their communication "axis" interact with each other to influence our overall mental wellness. Even more important, *Mental Fitness* also focuses on not just understanding this three-brain relationship but on practical approaches to act on this relationship to improve how we feel and perform.

PART 1

THE GUT-HEART-
BRAIN AXIS

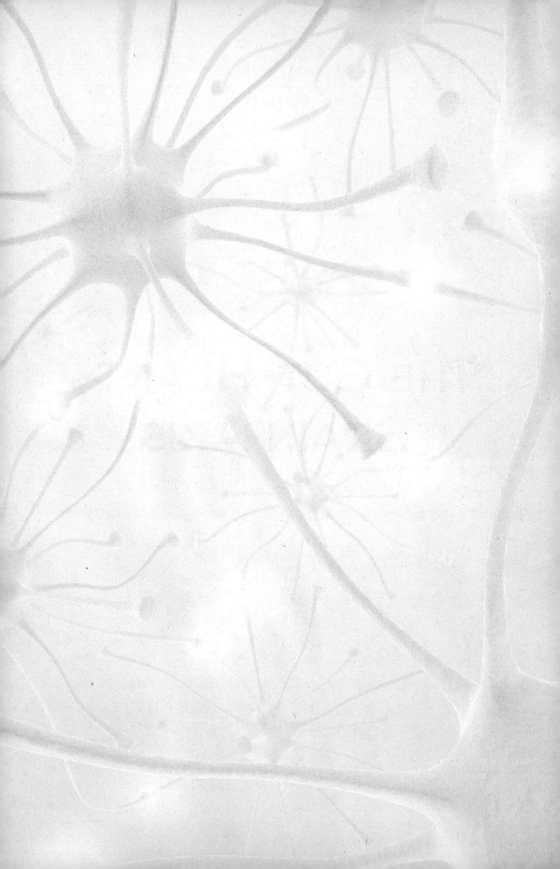

CHAPTER 1

THE BRAIN

The human brain is perhaps the most complicated "machine" that has ever existed. With more than eighty-six billion neurons that create more than one hundred trillion connections (synapses), the human brain is more highly networked and intricately connected than the entire global internet. The estimated memory capacity of the human brain is about one petabyte (one million gigabytes) and roughly equivalent to that of the entire World Wide Web. Quite simply, the three-pound organ in our head is the most complex object in the known universe. It's capable of astonishing feats of creativity, logic, computation, problem-solving, and understanding—each of which can be improved and optimized to help us lead our best lives.

The human brain is larger than expected for a mammal our size (by about seven to eight times) but still only about one-third the weight of an elephant's brain and about one-fifth that of a whale. Rather than overall brain size, a more important metric for what makes a human brain so special is not just the sheer number of total neurons but especially the sixteen billion cortical neurons—those packing the outermost wrinkly layer of the brain called the cerebral cortex. It's the cortex that enables humans to develop complex logic and excel at problem-solving, strategy formation, planning, creativity, and adaptability.

Our brain is composed of at least seventy-five different types of cells—not only electrical-impulse-conducting neurons but also non-electrical cells called glial cells that are at least as numerous as neurons. Smaller glial cells called microglial cells are part of the brain's immune system, roaming the brain and gobbling up foreign material that could damage neurons. Astrocytes are a type of glial cell that helps modulate the neuronal environment by controlling levels of neurotransmitters and helping to repair neuron damage. Astrocytes are also involved in the "pruning" of old or disused neuronal connections, which is a direct approach to the "brain plasticity" that enables our brains to grow and change both their structure and function in response to our experiences. In addition to the vast array of brain cells, there are also spaces between the cells—chambers called ventricles that produce the fluid that bathes all of our brain cells. We make about a pint of this cerebrospinal fluid every day, which cushions the brain, carries nutrients, and washes away toxins to keep the brain in good working order.

All of the brain cells can be broadly divided into gray matter (the main bodies of neurons) and white matter (the five hundred miles of fibers down which they send signals). The characteristic deep folds of gray matter, which give our brains a walnut-like appearance, bring the neurons closer together and enable a much faster speed of processing and communication between neurons. Research shows us that smarter people have more highly folded brains and, even better, that anyone can actively increase both our individual folding patterns and enhance the connectivity between different brain regions with directed learning. We all can get smarter and grow our brains—even into old age. This idea of being able to actively change our brains is called "brain plasticity" to denote the brain's malleability in improving its efficiency of conducting nerve signals through the neuronal network as well as changing the "shape" of the brain into a new and improved structure.

We can think of our brains as being divided into two "sides"(left and right) and also into two "layers" (top and bottom). Many people think of themselves as having a specific personality type dominated by being either "left-brained" (rational, logical, and analytical) or "right-brained" (creative, artistic, and free-spirited). In truth, this is mostly a myth, and research tells us that we're always using our whole brain. That said, most people process language in the left hemisphere, whereas our emotions are handled on the right. This fact led to the misconception that our left side handled *only* logical thinking and our right side processed *only* emotions, but it's actually much more nuanced than that. For example, although our left hemisphere produces complex speech, the right side allows us to understand the emotional and abstract aspects of those words. Creative thought, rather than being confined to just the left side, actually activates a widespread network of cells across both hemispheres.

Rather than thinking of our brains as being divided by left and right (which they are structurally), newer research is suggesting that a top/bottom distinction makes more sense when we consider how the brain functions. The top regions are involved in formulating and carrying out plans and adjusting them as we go based on new information and experiences. The bottom regions are largely concerned with processing inputs from our emotions and senses (including our gut and heart—more on that later), classifying objects, and giving meaning to feelings and events. Here again, we all use our entire brain all the time, but each of us to some extent is more top-brained or bottom-brained, each with associated benefits and drawbacks. For example, a more top-brained person might be a creative go-getter but may struggle from an inability to update plans based on new information and changing situations (entrepreneurs are often like this—jumping out of the plane and building the parachute on the way down). Likewise, bottom-brained types may excel at the planning stages of a project, coming up with a million great concepts and ideas, but they may be reluctant or unable to pull the trigger on moving the project forward in a meaningful way. Just as targeted learning and experiences can improve the connections between our left/right hemispheres, we can also improve the connections between our top/bottom brain regions—and in doing so, we can enhance our effectiveness across multiple types of intelligence.

Top Brain—also known as our "logical" brain—includes the neocortex, which makes up about 80 percent of brain mass and is instrumental in our ability as humans to create, execute, and monitor plans:

➤ Frontal lobe—problem-solving, complex thinking, decisions

➤ Prefrontal cortex—planning complex behavior

➤ Motor cortex—planning and executing movement

➤ Parietal lobe—perception and integration of sensory information

Bottom Brain—also known as our "primitive" brain—operates mostly on a subconscious emotional level to help us classify and interpret emotional information:

➤ Temporal lobe—hearing (auditory cortex), processing sensory information into memories

➤ Occipital lobe (includes visual cortex)—visual processing

➤ Hippocampus—memory

➤ Amygdala—regulates emotions and especially fear/stress reactions

➤ Nucleus accumbens—controls the release of dopamine (neurotransmitter of motivation and reward)

➤ Cerebellum—controls muscle function

➤ Pituitary gland—releases beta-endorphins (decrease pain), oxytocin (increases feelings of trust), adrenocorticotropic hormone (for cortisol release by the adrenals), and growth hormone

➤ Hypothalamus—the first node of the hypothalamic-pituitary-adrenal axis (HPA axis) that controls our stress response system, releases corticotropin-releasing hormone, which stimulates the pituitary gland to release adrenocorticotropic hormone, which stimulates the adrenal glands to release adrenaline (epinephrine) and cortisol

Research has shown that our ability to solve unique problems (fluid intelligence) is related to both the volume of gray matter in the frontal lobe and the amount of white matter connections between the two halves of the prefrontal part of the brain. Human intelligence is also related to the fact that our brains never fully power down (until death); they're always displaying certain levels of activity, even while we sleep. The brain regions that are most active during rest are referred to as the "default mode network," and it is these regions that are most active when we're daydreaming and when our attention is otherwise switched off. The default mode network is thought to be responsible for our ability to mull over past experiences and speculate about the future and also for the spark of insight that often comes after "sleeping on" a particular decision. During sleep, our brain is a hive of activity, including clearing out of toxic metabolites, regulating hormone levels, and conjuring dreams, which are thought to engage the default mode network during REM sleep to help us file away experiences for later recall (learning) and simulate new behaviors that can help us during waking life (insight).

Just as our brain is divided into conscious and subconscious "sections" that we refer to as the central nervous system, the rest of our "peripheral" nervous system that reaches out to every corner of our body is also divided into sections that can operate independently of conscious direction from the brain.

Our Unconscious Nervous System

Have you ever wondered how you digest food (without consciously deciding to do so), why you sweat or get short of breath when stressed, or why in tense situations you might feel nauseous or have to visit the toilet? All of these functions and more are controlled by your "unconscious" or autonomic nervous system (ANS). Your ANS is a branch of the nervous system that regulates your internal organs, heart, stomach, glands, smooth and cardiac muscles—mostly things that you cannot consciously control. While you might not know it, this system is constantly engaged and unceasingly changing millisecond by millisecond to help you best adapt to what's going on in the world around you.

To break it down even further, the autonomic system has two parts—the sympathetic nervous system (SNS) and parasympathetic nervous system (PNS)—that work inversely, but in a (mostly) coordinated fashion. The SNS, more commonly known for its fight-or-flight characteristics, helps regulate your stress response as part of the HPA axis described earlier (and which we'll come back to later).

Today, most of us are swimming in a sea of stress. Whether it's caused by work, school, peers, loved ones, or something else, we all at some point experience it. Stress can be defined as "a state of mental, emotional, or physical strain or tension resulting from adverse or very demanding circumstances," and for many of us, this is our default state. Interestingly, our bodies have the same physiological response to "nonimmediate stress"—such as dropping your iPhone or seeing you have ten missed calls from Mom—as we would to a life-or-death survival situation. These responses result from neurotransmitters and hormones, chemical messengers that travel throughout our body sending signals to help communicate between different organs and systems. At any moment of the day or night, we might have fifty-plus hormones and neurotransmitters at work regulating everything from heart rate, blood pressure, body temperature, water retention, sleep cycles, cellular growth, glucose levels, and so on.

Conversely, while the SNS is there to "rev" our engine, the PNS works to help calm us—what we refer to as "rest and digest." It helps in maintaining our body and conserving energy, digesting food, reproduction, waste excretion, and fighting infection. A set of twelve cranial nerves control sensory and motor functions throughout the body. Most important is the vagus nerve (the tenth cranial nerve, named after the Latin word for "wandering" and the root of the word *vagrant*) because it innervates many tissues, including connecting from your first brain to your second brain (gut) and third brain (heart) as well as to other important organ systems, such as the lungs and the adrenal glands. As a vital part of the ANS, the vagus nerve coordinates communications among our three brains (think of "gut feelings" and "trusting your heart"). You can actively engage "vagal tone" with techniques as simple as deep breathing, which almost immediately calms an overactive stress response (more on that later).

The SNS and PNS systems work together to keep your body in balance. Rather than rivals, imagine a scale or a seesaw with SNS ("rev") on one side and PNS ("calm") on the other, constantly trying to shift toward equilibrium. Your autonomic system is constantly making adjustments, such as changing your body temperature, slowing your heart rate, and sending extra blood to a particular area of your body in order to achieve this equilibrium, known as homeostasis. Without it, you would be an irrational mess of emotions and hormones. You wouldn't be able to regulate when you are full or hungry or fight back when something threatens you. The autonomic system plays an important role, holistically, when it comes to your mental and physical well-being.

All of this brain activity and signaling "ability" of our neurons and various brain regions relies on specialized chemical messengers called neurotransmitters. There are more than two hundred known chemical messengers in the body, allowing a wide range of cell-to-cell communication and affecting virtually every aspect of our daily lives—our mood, energy levels, mental focus, stress levels, pain perception, immune function, creativity, motivation, and many other aspects of our overall physical health and mental well-being.

KEY NEUROTRANSMITTERS INVOLVED IN MENTAL WELLNESS		
NEUROTRANSMITTER	PRIMARY FUNCTION	WHEN SUBOPTIMAL
GABA (gamma-aminobutyric acid)	Relaxation	Tension Anxiety Insomnia
Acetylcholine	Muscle Contraction	Fatigue Cravings/Addiction Brain Fog

Dopamine	Motivation/Reward	Fatigue
		Depression
		Lack of Enthusiasm/ Enjoyment (Anhedonia)
Serotonin	Mood/Happiness	Depression
Norepinephrine	Focus/Alertness	Brain Fog
		Attention Deficit
Epinephrine (Adrenaline)	Alertness/Vigilance	Brain Fog
		Fatigue
Histamine	Stress Response	Irritability
	Immune Support	Frequent Colds/Flu/ Allergies
Oxytocin	Feelings of Connection/ Trust	Social Disconnection
		Loneliness/Isolation
Brain-Derived Neurotrophic Factor (BDNF)	Neuronal Growth/ Survival	Memory Problems
	Brain Plasticity	Brain Atrophy
		Dementia
Endorphins	Analgesic (Pain Control)	Pain
Endocannabinoids	Neuromodulation	Pain
	Regulate Homeostasis (Balance)	Memory Problems
		Tension/Anxiety
		Insomnia

Is our brain really in charge?

With this level of complexity across neurons, synapses, brain regions, and neurotransmitters, you might think (as almost everyone has for centuries) that the brain is the ultimate "decider," meaning that the brain exclusively determines our thoughts and our behaviors, that it alone governs our emotions and moods, and that it largely "runs the show" when it comes to how we think and perform. If you thought all that about your brain, you'd certainly be in good company—but you would be wrong.

There is no doubt that our brains are intimately involved in how we think, how we feel, and how we behave, but the brain in our head is just one of several "brains" in the human body—and just one part of the larger brain-body connection. Gut feelings and trusting your heart are more than just turns of phrase; they have been part of our collective vocabulary for centuries, because we could "feel" these sensations even while we could not fully understand or explain why. Science now tells us that the microbes in our intestines and the electrical signals from our heart are "read" by the brain and can dramatically influence our mood and behavior as well as our mental and physical health. As such, the chemical signals emanating from our gut bacteria (microbiome) and the electrical field generated by our heart can also be thought of as "neurotransmitters" that signal the brain in our head to function and perform in certain ways. This emerging concept of our "three brains" is fundamentally changing how we think about mental fitness and human performance, and the new science is providing us with many additional tools to help us flourish in our increasingly stressful world.

CHAPTER 2

GUT BRAIN
(AND MICROBIOME)

More than two thousand years ago, the ancient Greek physician and father of modern medicine, Hippocrates, declared that "all disease begins in the gut"—which, up until recently, was often viewed as a quaint and outdated idea. Aside from conditions with observable "gut symptoms," such as stomach ulcers, IBS, and Crohn's disease, most health-care practitioners would not think much about the gut having health impacts in other parts of the body.

However, consider that we feel "butterflies" in our stomach when we fall in love or when we're nervous. We have a "gut feeling" about decisions we're wrestling with. Our stomach "growls" when we're hungry, and we feel "sick to our stomach" when we're stressed out. Many of us also know that when our gut is "off," we simply don't feel our best and vice versa: when we're stressed or depressed, our gut also suffers.

These and many other examples demonstrate the close connection between the brain in our head (our "thinking" brain) and the "second brain" in our gut (what we also call our "sensing" brain). We often say that we make decisions on the basis of gut feelings. Scientific studies have shown how a physical sensation, such as feeling nauseated, predictably leads to psychological effects, such as making us judge certain moral violations more harshly. We now consider the gut to be a "sense" organ, with the ability to detect sensations internally within our bodies and externally within our environment (including within social interactions).

From an anatomical perspective, we know that the gut lining has distinct "taste" receptors distributed throughout the entire gastrointestinal tract and is responsible not only for detecting incoming nutrients, toxins, and pathogens but also relaying that information to our brains. The gut contains more than five hundred million neurons to independently coordinate the process of digestion (without input from the brain) and more than four pounds of bacteria (the microbiome), which influence every organ in the body, including the brain.

A wealth of studies in mice show that changing the bacteria in the gut can change behavior related to introversion/extraversion, depression/ anxiety, and obesity/leanness. In humans, consuming fermented foods (yogurt) and dietary supplementation with specific strains of probiotic bacteria can have a profound effect on resting brain activity and behavioral/emotional responses to stressful events. Indeed, newer research is showing that certain types of gut bacteria are associated with depression, and emerging evidence suggests that a wide range of neurological conditions such as autism and Alzheimer's may originate in the gut. For example, in Parkinson's disease, alpha-synuclein fibers—a hallmark of the disease—seem to appear first in the gut, up to a decade before spreading to the brain (perhaps via the vagus nerve). In epilepsy, changes to the gut microbiome and the signals they send may explain why high-fat "keto" diets can prevent certain seizures in some people. These recent findings around the tens of trillions of bacteria in our gut and the universe of bioactive compounds and metabolic activity have led to the concept of "psychobiotics"—medicines that target the microbiome to improve our mental health.

From the perspective of size, our gut brain—what we call the "enteric nervous system" (ENS)—is only about 1/200 as large as our head brain (around five hundred *million* neurons in the ENS versus about one hundred *billion* in the brain). But what our gut brain lacks in sheer volume it makes up for in terms of neurotransmitter production. We typically think of neurotransmitters like serotonin and dopamine as mood chemicals that are produced in the brain—and they are, but only to a point. Up to 95 percent of the body's serotonin (the neurotransmitter of "happiness") is made in the gut. Likewise, the gut makes up to 70 percent of our dopamine (for motivation), along with the majority of our norepinephrine (for focus), GABA (for relaxation), and many others.

In addition to its production of neurotransmitters, the gut also contains more than 70 percent of our immune system (which helps our brains communicate with each other—more on that in coming chapters) and is home to the nearly one hundred trillion bacteria that make up our microbiome, which in many ways is like having an internal on-demand natural pharmacy.

What Is the Gut Microbiome?

The term *microbiome* refers to the trillions of bacteria, viruses, fungi, and other microscopic creatures that inhabit our gastrointestinal tract. Before you get too grossed out, consider that these inhabitants (mostly bacteria) have coevolved with us for millions of years—and have inhabited the planet for hundreds of millions of years longer than humans have even been around. Rather than thinking of bacteria as enemies, we need to think of them as friends and allies in optimizing our health and well-being.

While it is difficult to get a precise number of the total bacterial count, studies have suggested that our microbiome contains between twenty to one hundred trillion bacteria (which can change during the course of life, based on age and health status). Compare that to the number of cells in the human body (about ten trillion) or the number of neurons in the human brain (about one hundred trillion) and you can appreciate that we're dealing with a large number of bacteria. To give you a visual comparison, whatever number you choose for total bacterial count in the microbiome, it's many times more than the number of stars in the Milky Way, which is somewhere between two hundred billion and four hundred billion stars. Even more mind-boggling is that the ten million plus bacterial genes in the microbiome outnumber our own genetic diversity by a factor of more than one hundred times—which means that more than 99 percent of the genes in our bodies are microbial. These microbial genes can regulate how our human genes function, which can modulate our risk for a variety of diseases.

Probiotics, Prebiotics, and Fermented Foods

Once you know that the bacteria in your gut have such a major impact on your mental wellness and physical health, you're likely to be interested in supporting the healthiest microbiome that you can. Often, this means looking to dietary supplements, such as probiotics that provide beneficial bacteria as a means to improve gut health. On a positive note, a number of very good research studies in humans have shown that probiotic supplements can have significant benefits for many aspects of mental wellness (such as depression, anxiety, stress, and more) and physical health (like immune support, inflammatory balance, constipation, diarrhea, and gas/bloating). On a less positive note, the benefits of probiotic supplements are "strain-specific," meaning that certain strains of bacteria deliver certain specific benefits (and not other benefits), so you need to know the strain to understand its effects—and the vast majority of commercially available probiotic products don't disclose the strains in the formula. This is a problem. You would never buy a multivitamin that just said "vitamins" on the label, so why would you buy a probiotic that simply listed bacteria by the genus (such as "*Lactobacillus*") and species (such as "*rhamnosus*") without knowing the strain (such as "R0011," which tells you that this particular strain of *Lactobacillus rhamnosus* has benefits for reducing stress).

Before we go too much further, let's define what we mean by probiotic. Probiotics are defined by the WHO as "live microorganisms which when administered in adequate amounts confer a health benefit on the host." Probiotics (the actual bacteria) are not to be confused with prebiotics, which are defined by the International Scientific Association for

Probiotics and Prebiotics as "a substrate that is selectively utilized by host microorganisms conferring a health benefit." So probiotics are the bacteria, and prebiotics are their food (such as fiber) or something that improves their health (such as phytonutrients).

Dietary supplements of certain probiotics or prebiotics (or a combination of the two, often called "synbiotics") can provide a wide range of mental wellness and physical health benefits, but not all bacteria are probiotics (unless they have a demonstrated health benefit), nor is all fiber considered prebiotic (unless it is used by the bacteria to confer a health benefit).

Typical dietary sources of prebiotics include fruits and vegetables such as whole grains, oatmeal, beans, bananas, asparagus, leeks, and chicory. Prebiotic fiber in our diet arrives undigested to the large intestine (colon) where it nourishes the bacteria in our microbiome and increases the population and activity or our "good" bacteria, including *Lactobacillus* and *Bifidobacterium*. Unfortunately, the extreme lack of total fiber and especially prebiotic fiber in the Western diet is known to lead directly to the steep increase in inflammatory diseases, cancer, obesity/ diabetes, depression/anxiety, and other "modern" diseases of the twenty-first century. Supplementation with prebiotic fiber has been shown to reduce stress, anxiety, and depression as well as increase stress resilience and cognitive function. In fact, studies of specific prebiotic fibers such as beta-galacto-oligosaccharides (B-GOS) and galactomannan have even shown improvements in social behavior in cases of autism spectrum disorder, which is a classic example of a condition defined by disruptions in the microbiome and entire gut-brain axis.

Probiotics, whether consumed as supplements or in fermented foods—think yogurt, kefir, kombucha—exert their health benefits through a variety of pathways, including interacting with our resident microbiome bacteria and intestinal lining (epithelium). Through these interactions, and depending on the bacterial strains, ingested bacteria have been shown to improve metabolism (helping blood sugar balance and cholesterol levels); immunity (fighting colds/flus and allergies);

and hormone balance (including estrogen/testosterone balance, thyroid function, and cortisol sensitivity) and even slow certain markers of the aging process (like inflammation/oxidation).

Perhaps the most intriguing effect of probiotics and prebiotics is their ability to directly (and quickly) modulate brain physiology, leading to improvements in mental wellness. Increasingly, probiotics and prebiotics are being viewed as not just natural approaches to help us feel better but also as interventions that can actually help us perform better with improved neurotransmission (faster thinking, greater creativity, sharper focus), increased neurogenesis (protection of existing brain cells, growth of new neurons, increased neuronal connectivity), and reduced neuroinflammation (better memory, reduced risk for dementia and Alzheimer's disease). Indeed, human clinical trials have shown that specific probiotic strains (*Lactobacillus helveticus* R0052 and *Bifidobacterium longum* R0175) reduce depression, anxiety, and stress. Rodent studies using the same strains have indicated enhanced protection of brain regions typically damaged by chronic stress and during the aging process (hypothalamus, hippocampus, amygdala). Since we can't dissect human brains after probiotic supplementation studies, researchers are beginning to use functional magnetic resonance imaging (fMRI) techniques to show how "psychobiotic" bacteria can improve brain activity, including fear responses in the amygdala, connectivity in the prefrontal cortex, and activity in the hypothalamus. These are directly related to measures of brain performance and cognitive ability.

In addition to probiotics (the bacteria) and prebiotics (the fibers that they use for fuel), there are the newer concepts of phytobiotics, postbiotics, and protobiotics. Phytobiotics describe non-fiber plant compounds (such as polyphenols) that can change the structure and function of the microbiome. Postbiotics describe the bioactive compounds (such as short-chain fatty acids, or SCFAs) that are produced by the microbiome and have signaling effects across the entire gut-heart-brain axis. Finally, protobiotics—where "proto" means primary or first, as in "prototype"—describe an advanced sort of synbiotic that combines pro-pre-post-phytobiotics into a unified approach to whole-body health that starts in the gut.

What Is the Microbiome Doing?

When studying the important role of the microbiome in gut-brain axis function, we need to answer two very important questions: "Who is there?" (what bacteria are present—or absent) and "What are they doing?" (what fuels they are using and what metabolites they are producing). The last decade has seen an explosion in the field of bioinformatics, where computer algorithms are used to describe biological principles. These tools include many of the DNA-analysis techniques developed as part of the Human Genome Project, completed in 2003, that decoded our around 23,000 human genes. Since there are ten to one hundred times more bacterial genes in the microbiome (compared to our human genome), the Human Microbiome Project (launched in 2007) has had to develop entirely new analytical techniques to assess DNA, RNA, and a wide range of bacterial metabolites so we can begin to understand what specific strains are present and what they are producing (good and bad) that may influence human health and well-being. Perhaps most interesting of all, when it comes to studying our microbiome, is that our bacterial genes clearly influence the expression of our human genes. While we cannot change our human genetic profile, we can rapidly and dramatically change our microbiome. Thus, we can change its influence on our health and future disease risk.

When we use genetic analysis techniques in the lab, we gain a perspective on the total numbers of bacteria present ("absolute abundance"), their numbers in relation to other species/strains ("relative abundance"), similarities/differences between bacteria present ("diversity"), and resistance to change/stress and ability to bounce back to normal ("robustness" and "resilience"). All of these ways of looking at our microbiome are important because they provide different but interrelated perspectives on the overall ecology of our microbiome balance. Looked at from these multiple perspectives, our microbiome is a rich and complex ecosystem that is in a constant state of ebb and flow and flux across our life span and health span.

Early Microbiome

Most research suggests that the human gastrointestinal tract is first colonized by bacteria at birth when the baby passes out of the birth canal and is inoculated with the mother's vaginal microbiome. Maternal factors such as diet, stress, sleep patterns, metabolism (influencing obesity/diabetes), medication use, immune activation, and many others are known to influence the baby's mental and physical health outcomes—many of which seem to be mediated via changes in the microbiome. It is becoming increasingly clear that the early microbiome plays a critical role in ensuring proper development of the infant's immune system, brain, and blood-brain barrier.

From birth and continuing for at least the first three years of life, the baby's microbiome becomes more and more diverse, especially after weaning and when solid foods are introduced. Prior to weaning, research has shown a negative impact on microbiome diversity and robustness from Cesarean section delivery (versus vaginal delivery) and formula feeding (versus breastfeeding). Babies delivered via C-section tend to have a microbiome predominated by bacteria that resemble skin species, and formula-fed babies miss out on the rich source of breastmilk-derived prebiotic sugars (oligosaccharides), so they tend to have a less diverse microbiome. Both C-section and formula-fed babies also tend to have higher risk for developing immune-involved conditions later in life, including type 1 diabetes, asthma, eczema, and allergies—suggesting that our early-life microbiome has long-lasting health implications (unless we intervene to restore balance). Even in very early life, the microbiome can be influenced by other factors, including birth location (hospital versus home), antibiotic use, stress, pet ownership, city/country residence, and many others that have been linked in research studies to long-term outcomes such as behavioral temperament (whether a person tends toward tense/calm and happy/sad, for example), brain connectivity (likelihood of conditions like autism and ADHD), and metabolism (odds of being obese or lean).

Teenage Microbiome

Adolescence is undoubtedly a time of great physical change and psychological disruption. Hormones fluctuate, bones grow, muscles develop, and bodies change shape. But as much as our bodies are undergoing dramatic shifts during our teenage years, our brains are experiencing even more changes in functional connectivity and physical reshaping. The teenage brain undergoes changes in total volume in various regions (some of which continue into our early twenties) and in connectivity between those areas. In terms of microbiome balance, the teenage years appear to be characterized by a gradual shift from the rapidly changing early childhood period to a more stable adult microbiome—getting slightly more diverse and slightly more robust year by year. You might think of the microbiome during the teenage years in terms of a consolidation period where the rule is "don't screw it up." Unfortunately, there are lots of factors that can screw it up!

Studies have shown that stress (including inadequate sleep), poor diet, sedentary lifestyle, and antibiotic usage can have dramatic and long-lasting detrimental effects on virtually all aspects of microbiome balance, which can lead to heightened depression/anxiety and reduced levels of hormones (including oxytocin involved in empathy and BDNF involved in brain growth). It's not an overstatement to expect the typical American teenage experience of high stress, inadequate sleep, processed food diet, low physical activity, and antibiotics for every sore throat to lead to high schools (and colleges) filled with stressed/depressed/anxious students who are also disengaged and unmotivated. Indeed, this is precisely what we would predict based on the latest studies of the microbiome-gut-brain axis.

Aging Microbiome

As depressing as it sounds, the United Nations defines "older persons" as anyone over the age of sixty! At this age (and much earlier if you're not careful), we see the signs of aging as what we as scientists would describe as "a slow progression of deterioration in homeostatic mechanisms and accumulation of dysfunction." In other words, we get less good at maintaining balance (homeostasis), and we start to break down as a result of being out of balance. We can measure these imbalances and inefficiencies right down to the cellular and genetic level, where we can observe mitochondrial dysfunction, stem cell exhaustion, cellular senescence, oxidative stress, depressed autophagy, decline in growth factors, dysregulated immunity, neurotransmitter imbalances, disrupted nutrient signaling, altered stress axis responsiveness, and many, many others. Aging is also associated with changes in gut physiology, including degenerative changes in the ENS and gut lining (also known as leaky gut), disruptions in acid/base balance such as hypochlorhydria (low stomach acid), SIBO (small intestine bacterial overgrowth), and altered gut motility (constipation/diarrhea, for example)—all of which can lead to or be the result of an aging gut microbiome.

Recent studies have suggested that "health span" (how well we maintain good health into our later years) is determined in large part by the resilience and robustness of our microbiome. Decreasing diversity of the microbiome has been linked to accelerated aging and age-related impairments such as frailty and "inflammaging," where uncontrolled inflammation is at the heart of virtually every disease process, including Alzheimer's disease, heart disease, diabetes, and cancer. We know that a diverse diet and regular physical activity, which unfortunately often decline in later life, can dramatically influence cognitive performance, physical well-being, mental outlook, and microbiome balance at any stage of life, but their effects seem to be exaggerated in older individuals. For example, studies in semi-supercentenarians (people 105 to 109 years of age) have shown that the more diverse the diet, the more diverse the microbiota, with greater abundance of species such as *Lactobacillus, Bifidobacterium,* and *Akkermansia* as well as reduce Firmicutes/Bacteroidetes ratio. Animal studies have shown that exchanges of microbiome patterns from younger to older individuals increased the longevity of the older group. It is becoming increasingly clear that the microbiome may not only determine our early gut-brain development but also our midlife behavior and performance as well as our late-life health and longevity—so keeping our bacteria healthy is vital at all stages of life.

Microbiome and Our Mood

It's clear that there are a lot of neurons in the ENS and there are a *lot* of bacteria in our microbiome, but what does that mean for how we feel in terms of our moods, our emotions, and our behaviors?

As far back as 1,700 years ago (the fourth century), doctors practicing traditional Chinese medicine (TCM) treated gastrointestinal problems such as food poisoning and diarrhea with a remedy known as "yellow soup," which scientists today would refer to as an "oral administration of human fecal suspension." (Yep—they ate poop.) Ancient Greek physicians, including Hippocrates and Galen, were known to link mental states such as "melancholia" (what today we would call depression) to "black bile" (physical disruptions) that were treatable with both human and animal feces. Ancient Egyptians had a remarkably well-organized medical system, including physicians who specialized in different ailments and used human and animal excrement for their healing properties, including to ward off bad spirits (which today we might view as emotional problems). More recently, fecal microbiota transplantations (FMT), which involve transferring fecal material from a healthy donor to a diseased recipient to alter microbiome balance, have been used successfully to treat gut infections such as C. diff (refractory *Clostridium difficile*) and experimentally in other conditions including IBS, inflammatory bowel disease (IBD), and autism.

A range of more modern experiments—from mouse studies to applying antibiotic medications to actually transferring bacteria from humans to animals—have all shown that bacteria can dramatically influence mood and behavior as well as produce long-lasting effects on brain development (including growth of new neurons, function and longevity of existing neurons, neurotransmitter balance, and many others). Even more intriguing is the growing list of human clinical trials showing how modulating microbiome balance, positively or negatively, can dramatically alter mental wellness and physical health.

Much of the early research on the gut-brain axis concerned the influence of the digestive tract (gut) on appetite and satiety (brain). These indicated that much of our appetite and cravings are signals that our brain receives from our gut (the actual tissue of the gut producing appetite hormones) and microbiome (the bacteria producing neurotransmitters and other signaling molecules). This early research has brought us to more recent studies showing how stress and inflammation can interfere with many of these signaling pathways (e.g., leading to depression, stress-eating, and cravings for comfort foods), while proactive interventions such as proper diet and probiotic/prebiotic supplements can support superior mental health and metabolism.

Our "Plastic" Brains and Genes

Neuroplasticity is the term used to describe the ability of the brain to organize and reorganize itself—to literally change shape ("plasticity")—in response to injury, disease, new situations, learning, experience, and influences from our second and third brains. This same phenomenon of tissue plasticity is observed across all parts of our dynamic gut-heart-brain axis, including right down to our genetic levels at our DNA, and we'll come back to it in more detail in future sections. For now, it's important to keep in mind that the signals that govern and direct plasticity are multidirectional, coming from and going to each of our brains in a coordinated fashion. For example, the microbiome synthesizes a variety of signaling molecules (such as SCFAs, neurotransmitters, B-complex vitamins, amino acids, and hormones) that can have direct effects on brain plasticity, including neurogenesis (growth of new brain cells), synaptogenesis (new connections between neurons), synaptic remodeling (strengthening/weakening those connections), and activity in various brain regions involved in learning, memory, mood, and behavior. These many aspects of microbiome mediated brain plasticity can be further influenced by external factors such as antibiotic use, immune activation, inflammatory balance, stress hormone exposure, gut integrity, physical activity patterns, and probiotic/prebiotic intake, among others.

In addition to the direct and indirect contact that microbiome cells can have with immune cells, peripheral nerves, and gut epithelial cells, the relationship between microbiota and our human genome is another mode of influence that our microbiome has on our brain (and our entire body). While the microbiome influence on our human genes does not change the gene itself, the epigenetics ("epi-" meaning "above" the gene) can determine whether a given human gene is expressed ("turned on") or not. Through a recently discovered pathway involving noncoding RNAs (microRNAs, or miRNAs), gut microbiota have been shown to regulate the expression of miRNA in the amygdala (fear center of the brain), offering us the potential to harness the power of our microbiome to improve mood states such as anxiety and potentially to treat a wide range of neuropsychiatric diseases.

Unbalanced Microbiome and Diseased States

As science has uncovered mystery after mystery concerning the microbiome and how it influences gut-brain axis signaling and ultimately our overall mental wellness and physical health, microbiome disruptions (dysbiosis) have also been implicated in a growing list of psychological and neurological diseases. Of particular note is that many of these gut-brain axis diseases are also related to imbalances in the HPA axis (hypothalamic-pituitary-adrenal) that regulates our response to and resilience against the many stressors that we face daily.

Autism spectrum disorder (ASD) is a classic disruption within several levels of the gut-brain axis, including microbiome dysbiosis, gut and digestive complaints (stomachaches, food intolerances, constipation/diarrhea), gut permeability (leaky gut), immune dysfunction, neurotransmitter imbalances, and deficits in sociability. ASD afflicts at least 1 in 68 children worldwide, with males about four times more commonly diagnosed. Several studies have shown consistent alterations in the microbiome of children with ASD, including a reduced abundance of beneficial *Bifidobacterium* and increased abundance of inflammatory *Clostridia*. Both microbiome transfer (FMT) and prebiotic supplementation (B-GOS) have led to increases in *Bifidobacterium* levels and improvements in both gastrointestinal and behavioral symptoms in ASD kids.

Depression

Depression is the leading cause of disability globally, and it has recently been clearly and consistently linked to imbalances in the microbiome and disruptions across the HPA axis and inflammatory signaling pathways that comprise the "axis" portion of our gut-heart-brain axis (more on that later). Across a wide range of human studies, there is a consistent observation of reduced levels of "good" bacteria, such as *Lactobacillus* and *Bifidobacterium*, as well as a general reduction in overall microbiome diversity and microbiome metabolites (such as neurotransmitters and SCFAs), accompanied by elevations in cortisol (stress hormone). Importantly, these disruptions appear to be meaningfully reversed with specific diets (like the Mental Fitness Diet) and targeted supplementation (using specific bacterial strains and specific structures of prebiotic fibers).

Anxiety

Anxiety and depression frequently go hand in hand and typically represent a classic chicken-or-egg scenario where one leads to the other in a vicious cycle that is difficult to break. Anxiety may also be a frequent hallmark symptom associated with chronic fatigue syndrome (CFS), fibromyalgia, addiction, ADHD, bipolar disorder (previously referred to as manic depression), and PTSD—and all have been shown to respond positively to the same types of antidepression diets and supplements that improve microbiome diversity and resilience.

Obesity

While certainly not a "psychological" condition in and of itself, obesity (along with diabetes) is known to cluster with depression, bipolar disorder, anxiety, and related conditions such as leaky gut. We know that the microbiome is a primary regulator of our appetite, cravings, and food intake, and rodent studies have shown repeatedly that obese/lean traits can be transferred readily between animals via microbiome transplants. These point to a logical link between the microbiome and our metabolism. Indeed, both animal and human studies have shown that a relative increase in Firmicutes and/or decrease in Bacteroidetes predisposes to weight gain and obesity while a drop on the F/B ratio is associated with future weight loss and leanness.

Dementia

Alzheimer's disease is the leading cause of dementia and the most common neurodegenerative disorder. The characteristic protein plaques that develop in the brain and lead to dysfunction and tissue destruction appear to be closely related to microbiome metabolism and immune system response across the gut-brain axis. One of the most interesting differences noted between Alzheimer's patients versus healthy subjects is in the microbiome F/B ratio, which has also been observed in obesity and diabetes, suggesting that similar interventions toward improving this ratio may enhance energy metabolism and ameliorate risk for dementia simultaneously.

Summary

It is now widely accepted in scientific communities, and increasingly making inroads into mainstream medicine, that our gut microbiome is vitally important for optimal development and function of our brain. A wide range of clinical studies are emerging on a daily basis, demonstrating the profound implications of our microbiome on our performance neurologically (brain function such as memory and cognition), psychologically (mood states such as stress, depression, and anxiety), and physiologically (the interaction between mental fitness and physical performance). Undoubtedly, it is still early in our understanding of the ultimate implications of the microbiome in determining our mental wellness and physical health, but indications hint at the potential for the microbiome to be the linchpin for effective personalized medicine approaches in the (very near) future.

Given the role that lifestyle choices such as diet, exercise, sleep, stress, and environmental exposures have in modulating microbiome balance and thus determining gut-heart-brain axis signaling, coming chapters will focus on steps you can take to mediate not just how you feel but also how you perform and how long you live with abundant health.

CHAPTER 3

HEART BRAIN

In chapter 1, we learned about the brain in our head—our thinking brain. In chapter 2, we learned about the "second brain" in our gut—our sensing brain. Now in this chapter, we'll learn about the "third brain" in our heart—our feeling brain.

You've undoubtedly heard many expressions that describe the importance of our heart to the broad range of human emotions and experiences. Here are some examples:

- Trust your heart
- Listen to your heart
- Follow your heart
- Broken heart
- Heart in your mouth
- Heart on your sleeve
- Know something "by heart"

- Heart isn't in it
- Heart of glass
- From the bottom of your heart
- My heart goes out to them
- Bleeding heart
- Eat your heart out

In many traditional medicine systems, including Chinese (TCM), Indian (Ayurveda), Japanese (Kampo), and Native American, the heart plays a central role as both the seat of the human spirit and a bridge between the body and mind. Ancient Greek philosophers such as Aristotle and physicians such as Galen believed that the heart, not the brain, was the center of human emotions. In more modern times, we have known since the 1950s about the linkage between heart function and emotional well-being—from studies showing the increased risk for depression in heart attack patients and the higher rate of heart problems among people with chronic stress and anxiety. In the early 1990s, the new scientific and medical discipline of "neurocardiology" started to describe how the heart can not only act independently of the brain but can actually communicate directly with the brain to determine many aspects of our mental wellness and physical performance. In fact, a variety of clinical case reports have described how heart transplant patients have taken on the feelings, memories, and personalities of their donors. One unique condition known as stress-induced cardiomyopathy results from intense exposure to physical or mental stress leading to weakness and damage to the heart muscle. Since cardiomyopathy can occur after severe emotional stressors such as grief and loss of a loved one, it is sometimes referred to as "broken heart syndrome" and further indicates the close connections between our heart and our emotions.

The heart contains approximately forty thousand neurons, which is a smaller number than the billions of neurons in our head brain and the millions of neurons in our gut brain but still a large enough collection to be a powerful center of receiving and transmitting information that can determine our mental and physical performance. In fact, by measuring the relationship between heart rhythms and brain waves (whether or not they are in resonance or coherence with each other), we are increasingly able to not merely "show" the relationship between heart function and performance but to improve both. This heart-brain axis is similar to the gut-brain axis discussed in the last two chapters and is based on the emerging idea that a more efficient heart generates signals that lead to a more positive mood state—so in addition to the cardiovascular benefits of a healthy heart, you get a bonus set of psychological benefits by bringing the head and the heart into coherence with each other.

How the Heart "Talks" to the Brain

The heart is able to produce its own hormones and neurotransmitters. Epinephrine (adrenaline) is associated with the fight-or-flight stress response. Oxytocin is associated with close emotional connections, such as love. Acetylcholine is associated with feelings of calmness and relaxation. But the majority of the heart's signals are electrical in nature, what we refer to as "heart rhythms." The heart can also produce and be influenced by a variety of cellular signaling molecules called cytokines, which are sort of a cross between hormones and neurotransmitters and are involved in immune system function and inflammatory balance.

Let's discuss the "chemicals" first and then the "rhythms" next, so we know how these different but complementary signals influence the heart-brain axis.

Inflamed Brains

When cytokines are out of balance, our immune system function may be underactive, which can lead to a higher incidence of infections such as cold/flu and certain cancers, or it may be overactive, leading to autoimmune conditions such as Hashimoto's thyroiditis, eczema, rheumatoid arthritis, and many others. Imbalanced cytokines result in a generally overinflamed state of metabolism, which is very bad for all three of our brains. Excess inflammation has been linked to elevated risk for problems for the brain in our head, including depression and Alzheimer's disease; higher incidence of problems for our gut brain, including IBS and other inflammatory bowel diseases (such as Crohn's disease); and greater predisposition for problems in our heart brain, including elevated risk for heart failure and heart attacks.

The word *inflammation* is derived from the Latin *inflammare*—meaning to "set on fire"—because an injury or infection is typically red, warm, and painful. Pain and inflammation are normal body processes. Without them, you would literally not be able to survive for very long. Pain is a signal to your body that damage is occurring and you need to stop doing whatever is causing that damage. Inflammation is a process controlled by the immune system that protects your body from invading bacteria and viruses, but this process also helps regulate heart function, blood flow, and many other vital processes. Maintaining a normal balance of pain signals and inflammation is critical to good health and vigor.

When this balance becomes disrupted, you experience more inflammation and increased pain, along with less flexibility and reduced mobility. When you have too much inflammation, this process, which is supposed to be *protecting* you, actually *causes* more and more damage. For example, an overactive inflammatory response is "catabolic," leading to accelerated tissue breakdown in all of the body's tissue including bone (leading to osteoporosis), cartilage (leading to arthritis), and muscles— even the heart. Inflammation is also involved in emotional balance and brain function because inflammatory cytokines can block the activity of neurotransmitters produced in any of our three brains. So when your body experiences too much inflammation, you simply don't feel happy. Instead, you feel mentally exhausted and burned out—the opposite of vigor.

The normal process of inflammation helps dismantle and recycle older tissues that have become damaged or worn out or that simply need repair. This process is called "turnover" or "normal inflammation," and it occurs when newer tissue replaces older tissue. Before the age of thirty or so, this normal turnover process is perfectly balanced; for every bit of tissue that is damaged and removed, another similar (or greater) bit is put in its place. This means that, under ordinary circumstances, you're always making your tissue stronger and more resilient. After about age thirty, however, the turnover process becomes somewhat less efficient year after year. This causes a very slight loss of healthy tissue; you continue to break down and to remove some tissue, but the amount of healthy tissue added back is just a little bit less than it should be. As you age, the turnover process becomes less and less efficient, and your body's ability to heal itself from injury is reduced. This imbalance in tissue turnover and the "normal inflammation" process is the primary cause of the loss of flexibility, vigor, and the various "-itis" diseases that people tend to encounter as they get older.

With aging, these normal repair mechanisms start to dwindle, and, ironically, the very inflammatory process that has been helping "turn over" older tissue into healthy new tissue can completely turn *on* you. That leads to physical problems with pain, mobility, and flexibility, and it also leads to mental problems associated with depression, sleep, energy, and stress resilience.

Let's keep in mind that not all inflammation is bad. As you've just learned, inflammation is part of the normal healing and turnover process for any tissue. But when you experience *too much* inflammation, things go awry. This is known as chronic inflammation, in which healing is suppressed and tissue destruction is accelerated. Your body simply cannot heal itself or stop the damage when inflammation gets out of control. To illustrate this point, think about the ocean crashing against a protective seawall. The seawall represents your tissues, and the ocean is your inflammatory process. Over time, that wall will become broken and weakened by the crashing waves and will need to be repaired to return to optimal functioning. If the pace of repair fails to keep up with the pace of destruction, then the seawall fails and the ocean comes rushing in. That's the equivalent of tissue destruction and dysfunction. You need to maintain the integrity of the seawall (your tissue) by keeping up with repair and maintenance, but you can't do that if the ocean is continually crashing down on you.

A plethora of scientific and medical evidence demonstrates how to use diet, exercise, and supplementation to "calm" the ocean (to reduce damage caused by excessive inflammation) and to accelerate tissue repair (to keep that seawall intact). It is all a question of balance. You want to maintain a normal level of inflammation so you can then maintain a normal pace of tissue turnover and thus retain healthy tissue, flexibility, and mobility. As soon as you get even a small amount of chronic inflammation, you see a little bit more tissue deterioration, leading to a little more inflammation and still more tissue breakdown. Once this vicious cycle of inflammation/damage has begun, it can be very difficult to stop it—unless you have a comprehensive plan to control inflammation through multiple health practices.

Chronic Inflammation

It may help you to think of chronic inflammation as you would a fire in an apartment building. Let's say you live in a twenty-story apartment building, which represents your body. Then a fire (inflammation) breaks out on the fifteenth floor, causing destruction (tissue damage) to the entire floor. But your penthouse apartment on the twentieth floor is fine. To put out the fire, you call in the firefighters (immune cells), which may cause a bit more damage by tearing down some walls and spraying water (cytokines, secreted by immune system cells), all in an effort to solve the bigger problem of putting out the fire. Let's now say that the fifteenth floor is a complete loss, while other floors suffer some repairable damage (water damage on the fourteenth floor and smoke damage on the sixteenth floor). The repair process begins on all three floors, with carpenters, painters, and other builders brought in to repair the damage. On floors fourteen and sixteen, where the damage is less severe, the repair process might be complete within a few weeks; but on the fifteenth floor, where the fire was concentrated and the damage was most severe, the repair process may take a year.

When a tissue is damaged—whether from infection, trauma, or unbalanced turnover—it releases signaling chemicals called cytokines. These cytokines are like flare guns, sending up a call for help that signals surrounding cells to jump into action to stop, or wall off, and repair the damage. The cytokines also call immune system cells (white blood cells) into the area to help clean up the damaged tissue. You have no doubt experienced the blood rush that leads to the recognizable redness, warmth, and swelling common to many injuries. As the white blood cells rush into the damaged area, they release more and more of their own inflammatory chemicals. This blast of inflammation is intended to cause even more tissue destruction as a way to either kill bacteria and viruses or to take away damaged tissue and set the stage for repair efforts to begin. As you can imagine, this part of the inflammatory process is supposed to be short term. If it were to continue without shutting down, you'd simply destroy your own tissue without ever rebuilding healthy tissue in its place. This "never shut down" scenario precisely describes the chronic inflammation and constant state of tissue destruction with which millions of Americans live their lives every day.

Unfortunately, chronic inflammation is not confined to the tissue in which it starts. Cytokines—such as those labeled IL-6, IL-8, and TNF-alpha—are able to leave the original site of inflammation. They can then travel in the blood to spread inflammatory signals through the blood vessels and into every tissue in the body, leading to metabolic diseases, such as obesity, diabetes, and depression, and to structural-damage diseases, such as Alzheimer's, Parkinson's, and arthritis. Because most of the cytokine molecules are produced by immune system cells, numerous prescription drugs attempt to control chronic inflammation by suppressing immune function. For example, our body's first line of defense is our "innate" immune system, which includes specialized cells such as macrophages and neutrophils that gobble up bacterial and viral invaders and also includes natural killer (NK) cells that identify and kill cancer cells. Each of these immune cell types produces inflammatory cytokines as a way to kill pathogens and protect us from infection and disease. The problem, of course, is that wholesale suppression of immune function to reduce inflammation also limits your body's ability to protect you from actual pathogens—so you're "protected" from chronic inflammation, but you may become more susceptible to infections and certain cancers. Not a great trade-off!

Chronic inflammation not only affects the way you feel on a daily basis and the level of vigor you experience, it also contributes to the development of serious health conditions, including heart disease and depression. Researchers probably know the most about the adverse effects of chronic inflammation when it comes to heart disease. Until about ten years ago, most cardiologists and other health experts believed that heart disease was a simple "plumbing" problem, with too much cholesterol clogging up blood vessels and leading to heart attacks. Unfortunately, the cause of heart attacks was later determined to be a little more complicated. Population studies showed that at least half of all heart attacks occurred in people with perfectly normal cholesterol levels. What scientists know now is that oxidative damage (by free radicals) is what allows cholesterol to become "sticky" in the first place and to start plugging blood vessel linings with plaque deposits. Chronic inflammation, therefore, seems to be the "trigger" that causes those deposits to rupture and create a blockage in the heart, leading to a heart attack. The degree of chronic inflammation throughout the body can be measured by blood levels of a protein called "C-reactive protein" (CRP). CRP is produced in the liver, with levels rising in direct proportion to inflammatory signals in the body. During times of active infection (acute inflammation), CRP levels may rise by a factor of one thousand to fifty thousand in response to the increased production of cytokines, such as IL-6, from macrophages. A CRP value of 3.0 mg/L is associated with a tripling of heart attack risk, while people with very low CRP levels (below 0.5 mg/L) rarely have any sign of inflammatory heart disease. You may have to push for it, but you can ask to have your CRP levels tested the next time you're in the doctor's office.

If the inflammation process is a multifaceted chain reaction of biochemical events, then shouldn't your approach to controlling inflammation also be multifaceted? Of course it should! This is one of the many ways in which synthetic single-action pharmaceutical drugs fail miserably. Drugs are a single molecule, a single chemical entity, that work on *one* biochemical mechanism, albeit in a very powerful way— sometimes too powerfully, leading to serious side effects. For example, nearly 10 percent of those who use NSAIDs (nonsteroidal anti-inflammatory drugs, such as ibuprofen to control pain and inflammation) will require hospitalization due to serious gastrointestinal toxicity (such as ulcers and stomach bleeding). Nearly two hundred thousand people are admitted each year to hospitals—and another twenty thousand *die* each year—as a direct result of complications due to the use of NSAIDs. This is a problem for our gut brain as well as for our heart brain and our head brain, because being overinflamed and overexposed to cytokine signals can lead to direct damage of our gut lining, accelerated damage to our heart tissue, and unbalanced signals (chemical and electrical) being sent to our brain.

Your Charged Heart

Signals from the heart can be measured as electrical rhythms with a device called an electrocardiogram (ECG), which are increasingly being built into various fitness applications such as watches, rings, and heart rate monitors. The signals may be generated directly by the heart and also arrive in the heart from organs throughout the rest of the body. From the heart, the signals travel to the brain through a network of nerves, including the vagus nerve (the same nerve that also carries many of the nerve signals from the gut to the brain). The areas of the brain that receive these signals are primarily "primitive" preverbal areas of the brain such as the thalamus, hypothalamus, hippocampus, and amygdala that "think" in terms of emotions such as love, fear, hunger, and desire rather than logical words and thoughts. This is one of the reasons that we "feel" something in our heart or "sense" something in our gut, but we can't really describe it in words or explain rationally why we're feeling one way or another—we just "know" it.

When we measure heart function, we can look at our heart rate (the number of beats per minute) and our blood pressure (the pressure generated by the blood within our blood vessels during each beat of our heart) and even the elasticity of our blood vessels as they bulge and recover with each surge of blood from each heartbeat. One of the most useful measures of heart health is called heart rate variability (HRV), which analyzes the milliseconds between each individual heartbeat. HRV as a measure is based on the idea that a healthier heart contains *more* healthy irregularities than an unhealthy or stressed heart, which contains *fewer* irregularities. A higher HRV is healthier and indicates a heart that is more stress resilient.

HRV is an indicator of the balance between the branches of the ANS that we covered in chapter 1. Recall that the PNS is like the calming brake that allows our nervous system to "rest and digest," while the SNS is the revving gas pedal activating our fight-or-flight response. HRV can be thought of as a measure between PNS and SNS balance, with a higher HRV indicative of a calmer, more resilient, and more efficient heart.

Let's say that your resting heart rate is sixty beats per minute. That doesn't mean that your heart beats like a clock at consistent one-second intervals. Rather, there is a slight variation among the intervals between your heartbeats. The interval between your successive heartbeats can be, for example, 0.75 seconds between a certain two beats and 1.25 seconds between another two. Even though the difference is measured in milliseconds, you can actually *feel* the difference in terms of your mood, energy levels, and stress resilience (in general, the longest intervals take place when you exhale, and the shortest intervals when you inhale). Our HRV can be influenced by a variety of stressors, including physical stress, such as exercise, dehydration, or infection, and psychological stress, including work, school, finances, and sleep quality. Recent research from our group has shown that improvements in heart efficiency (measured by HRV) are also related to improvements in overall mental wellness (better mood, less tension, higher energy levels). Later on, we'll discuss some of the practical steps you can take to improve health across all three brains.

When the body is in balance (homeostasis), the heart is able to receive, generate, and transmit signals along the same coherent wavelengths. And when these signals are in complete resonance (tone) across the gut-heart-brain axis, we feel our best, with high emotional well-being and ample stress resilience. In these harmonic states of resonance/coherence, we are most likely to experience positive emotions, such as joy, happiness, love, gratitude, and resilience. When these signals are out of balance, we are more likely to experience feelings of stress, tension, anxiety, fear, anger, fatigue, sadness, and confusion. Aside from just "feeling" good or bad, our heart rhythm patterns can also influence our immune system function and our overall physical health. For example, it is well known within the medical community that approximately 90 percent of all doctor visits are primarily related to stress, and nearly 80 percent of all drug prescriptions are for conditions related to stress (antidepressants, antianxiety, sleep, hypertension, and similar concerns). In addition, the development of depression within six months following a heart attack is a hallmark predictor of premature death, suggesting that "affairs of the heart" are telling us a lot more about the overall state of the body than just its role as a circulation pump.

Our Harmonic Heart

The heart has been recognized to play a vital role not only as a circulatory pump but also as part of a psychophysiological network as a generator and transmitter of system-wide information throughout multiple body systems, including the nervous system. Electrical input from the heart can dynamically influence homeostatic, cognitive, perceptual, and emotional processing in the brain, thus having the potential to affect myriad aspects of mood and behavior. Organ crosstalk between the brain and heart has been noted in stress-related cardiomyopathy syndromes, where damage in the heart leads to stress/depression in the brain, and in traumatic brain injury, where damage in the brain leads to stress in the heart. In these situations, assessments of HRV can be useful for gauging both the state of the heart (physical stress) as well as the state of the brain (psychological stress). Yoga has been used as an intervention to restore balance to heart-brain crosstalk through plasticity and stability of the autonomic nervous system to reduce anxiety levels and to improve heart rhythm (atrial fibrillation episodes), blood pressure, and many other aspects of the heart-brain axis. Studies have also shown that the nature of the heart-brain axis is bidirectional, where positive emotional states may improve the function of both the cardiovascular and immune systems.

Because the gut-heart-brain axis is connected via the vagus nerve, activating this nerve with breath work can be an extremely simple, yet effective, way to reset heart-brain coherence and directly counteract feelings of stress and replace them with feelings of calmness.

Box Breathing

➤ Inhale slowly through your nose to a count of 5.

➤ Hold your breath for a count of 5.

➤ Exhale slowly through your mouth to a count of 5.

➤ Hold your breath for a count of 5.

➤ Repeat three times (total of 60 seconds).

> **Note:** As you become a regular user of this technique, you can become a bit more advanced in your practice by directing your thoughts toward each of your brains. What do you think about this situation (head brain)? What do you sense about this situation (gut brain)? What do you feel about this situation (heart brain)?

You can use this simple box breathing technique any time you need to reduce tension, calm down, relax, or focus. I personally use it while standing in line, sitting in traffic, preparing for bed, or calming my nerves before starting a race or giving a presentation. It does more than just help reduce negative emotions; when you combine it with positive thoughts, you replace the negative with the positive. Studies have shown that such techniques can also help reduce chronic pain and accelerate postsurgical tissue healing.

CHAPTER 4

AXIS

How Do Our Brains "Talk" to Each Other?

Many pathways exist for our gut to communicate with our brain, from highly complex nerve networks to highly modifiable ("plastic") neuronal complexes to dozens of bioactive molecules produced by the microbiome, the gut lining, and the brain cells. Importantly, these signals are "multidirectional," meaning that they can carry signals from the gut and the heart "up" to the brain as well as from the brain "down" to the gut and heart. These myriad signals are part of a highly complex overlapping communication network that we broadly refer to as the "axis" (as in "gut-brain axis") that functions as a whole-body surveillance network to detect and respond to threats, maintain balance (homeostasis), and modulate resilience across every organ system in our bodies. This network includes our microbiome, gut lining, enteric nervous system, central nervous system, cardiovascular system, immune system, inflammatory cascade, endocannabinoid system, and endocrine system.

If it wasn't interesting enough to know that we have this highly complex communication network inside us, we're also learning how this network *changes* over time—actually changing its shape and structural organization in response to our environmental exposures, social interactions, and daily experiences. For example, our gut microbiome changes its makeup in response to diet, our heart changes its electrical patterns in response to stress, and our brain neurons change their patterns of connections in response to learning and experience. All these "structural" alterations result in "functional" changes that determine how we feel and perform. Because of all of these overlapping functions within our axis, it's vitally important for both mental wellness and physical health that we "sync" these signals in order to feel and perform at our best. Indeed, clinical studies have shown that improving the efficiency of axis signaling can significantly boost psychological vigor (and reduce burnout, depression, and fatigue) in addition to the direct enhancements that can be made within each of our three brains.

Choose the Shape of Your Brain

We refer to the ability of a tissue to change its shape as being "plastic"—as in "brain plasticity" and "neuroplasticity" (from the Greek word *plastos*, meaning "molded")—to indicate the amazing ability of the brain to modify its own structure and function following internal or external factors. We now understand that all three of our brains are plastic, which means that we can change them in a direction that optimizes their function and thus our own performance. This very same plasticity principle also occurs in our immune system, our nervous system, our endocrine (hormone) system, and our endocannabinoid system (ECS) as well as across the entire three-brain communication axis. All of these systems are modifiable at any age along our entire life span.

Nerves

Both the sympathetic and parasympathetic systems can affect circuitry in the ENS—the nervous system within the gut—resulting in changes in gut motility and thus in the rate of delivery of nutrients to the small intestine and colon. This directly influences nourishment of the microbiome, because the bacteria may have more or less time to access the fibers and phytonutrients on which they thrive. This affects microbiome metabolism and production of metabolites, including serotonin, dopamine, norepinephrine, and gamma-aminobutyric acid (GABA), which can further mediate the quality of the intestinal mucus layer and integrity of the gut epithelial lining. So something as simple as being stressed, sleep-deprived, or worried can transmit a cascade of nervous system signals that impact every point along the gut-brain axis.

One of the most important nerves within the gut-brain axis is the vagus nerve, which provides a direct connection between the gut and the brain. It's comprised of 80 percent afferent (sensory) and 20 percent efferent (motor) fibers. Afferent fibers send signals from the body (gut and heart) to the brain, while efferent fibers carry signals from the brain to the gut and heart. The vagus nerve is a primary route of communication from the body to the brain. We have known for several decades that activation of the vagus nerve (with electrical stimulation and/or with deep breathing) can reduce levels of inflammatory cytokines and alleviate psychological pain, gut pain, and chronic systemic pain in other parts of the body. In animal studies, vagal stimulation has been associated with direct changes in levels of norepinephrine, serotonin, and dopamine in brain regions associated with depression and anxiety.

Neurotransmitters

The ENS is also known to respond to specific bacterial strains, via the bacteria-derived SCFAs such as butyrate, neurotransmitters such as serotonin, and inflammatory mediators such as cytokines. Changes in each of these classes of molecules are realized as alterations in our stress resilience, motivation, and even decision-making. As indicated in earlier sections, the majority of our neurotransmitters are produced in the gut (for example, as much as 90 to 95 percent of our serotonin), so interventions aimed at improving mental wellness must include attention to microbiome balance for optimal effectiveness.

Because neurotransmitters are signaling molecules that carry information from one nerve to another nerve, when we think about how to best modulate and optimize neurotransmitter balance, we need to consider where the neurotransmitters are originating (in the gut) and where they are having their desired effects (in the brain) as well as how we might be able to make their transmission more efficient (across the axis). Even though we can enhance how our head brain "receives" neurotransmitter signals and can improve how our gut brain "produces" neurotransmitter signals, we also need to pay attention to how our axis "carries" those signals across the body. Think of this signaling network like your internet connection; you might have a high-definition video on one end and a super-fast computer on the other end, but if they are connected by a rusty wire, the video performance will suffer as compared to a connection over a high-speed fiber-optic line.

Cytokines

Cytokines are hormonelike compounds produced primarily by immune system cells. They are one of the primary ways that cells communicate with each other. The word is derived from Greek, where *cyto* means "cell" and *kinos* means "movement"—so cytokine signals move between cells. Some of the most important effects cytokines help regulate are immune function and inflammation. Some cytokines have specific names determined by their function, such as chemokines, adipokines (from adipose tissue or fat), interferons, tumor necrosis factors (involved in cancer regulation), lymphokines (produced by and acting on immune cells called lymphocytes), and others.

Hormones

Like cytokines, hormones are also signaling molecules and also named from a Greek principle denoting "movement" or "motion." There is a bit of scientific argument about differences between hormones and cytokines. For the purposes of our discussions, the main difference really comes down to where the two are produced and where they act. Cytokines are produced by individual cells (largely within the immune system) and mostly act "close to home" in a region of the body. By contrast, hormones are produced by a network of glands (the endocrine system) and act "far from home" to regulate organ functions across the entire body. For example, cortisol produced in the adrenal glands above our kidneys influence system-wide stress responses. Thyroid gland hormones are produced in our neck yet influence overall energy metabolism. Insulin produced in the pancreas in our abdomen regulates blood sugar levels in every tissue in the body. The "love hormone" oxytocin, produced in the hypothalamus in the brain and also in the heart, influences our social connections with people external to our individual selves. Reproductive hormones such as testosterone and estrogen are produced in their respective male/female organs and regulate myriad functions, including growth, development, reproduction, and mood.

In many instances, hormones aren't actually "doing the work" that they may be known for, but rather they're kicking off a chain of events resulting in a change in function of a tissue, organ, or system. For example, many hormones are produced by their gland of origin, are secreted into the bloodstream, travel to a target tissue, and stimulate the production of regulatory proteins, sometime directly and sometimes by activating genes.

When any hormones are out of balance (dysregulated), that imbalance can cause a cascading domino effect that spreads imbalances to other hormones. Once that happens, restoring balance can be a frustrating undertaking. For example, dysbiosis in the microbiome can damage the gut lining, leading to gut permeability, which can interfere with immune system signaling. That increases systemic inflammation, leading to "blocking" the signaling functions of many neurotransmitters. Blocked serotonin leaves us feeling sad, and blocked dopamine makes us lose motivation, while problems with thyroid hormone make us gain weight and cortisol issues leave us feeling tense. Imbalance leads to more and more imbalance—and more and more problems with how we feel and how we perform. Luckily, the opposite is also true. Balance leads to more and more balance, which leads to increasing levels of feeling better and performing at our peak potential.

Endocannabinoid System

The endocannabinoid system (ECS) is yet another complex biochemical communication system spread across the entire gut-heart-brain axis. The messenger molecules within the ECS are known as endocannabinoids ("cannabinoid" referring to the structure of the molecules and "endo-"

indicating that they are produced internally within the body). You may be familiar with the term *phytocannabinoids*. These plant-derived versions of the same cannabinoid structures produced in the body can be derived from hemp and other plants.

Cannabinoids, whether produced in the body (endo-) or extracted from plants (phyto-) can bind with cannabinoid receptors (CB1 and CB2) to help regulate homeostasis (balance) in many parts of the body. In many ways, cannabinoids are similar to cell-signaling molecules like cytokines and to tissue-regulating molecules like hormones, but the main function of cannabinoids and their signaling within the ECS is to monitor for signals of imbalance across our axis. Whenever an "imbalance" emerges, such as physical or mental pain, cannabinoids are produced, the ECS is activated, and homeostasis is restored (often easier said than done).

Lately, there is a lot of hype around hemp extracts as sources of "CBD" to cure all varieties of depression, anxiety, pain, insomnia, and stress. Unfortunately, the hype rarely lives up to the reality. CBD is an abbreviation for "cannabidiol"—just one of more than one hundred phytocannabinoids found in hemp and other plants, such as chocolate, vanilla, peppers, and some spices. CBD from hemp is different from THC (tetrahydrocannabinol), the psychoactive cannabinoid responsible for the "high" in marijuana-derived products. Research has shown that cannabinoids have superior activity in regulating homeostasis when introduced as a blend (several cannabinoids) than when introduced in isolation (as a single cannabinoid)—what is often referred to as the "entourage effect." As such, it is logical that pure CBD extracts are unlikely to have the broad signaling effects needed across the ECS to adequately restore homeostasis when we're out of balance.

The primary endocannabinoid produced in our body is anandamide (also known by its chemical name arachidonoyl ethanolamine, or AEA). Anandamide is naturally derived from arachidonic acid (an omega-6 fatty acid) and ethanolamine (a key structural component of nerve cell membranes). It serves as a neurotransmitter within the ECS. The name "anandamide" is derived from the ancient Sanskrit word *ananda,* which means "joy" or "bliss," so AEA is often referred to as the "bliss molecule" because it helps reduce sensations of pain (mental and physical) to help you feel better.

Unfortunately, we can't take AEA as a supplement, because it gets broken down quickly by the fatty acid amide hydrolase enzyme (FAAH) back into its component parts (arachidonic acid and ethanolamine). Though we can't really "boost" production of AEA to help us feel better, we might be able to slow its breakdown by inhibiting FAAH. This is why many pharmaceutical companies are pursuing anti-FAAH compounds as a new class of antidepressants and painkillers, based on the idea that if you reduce the breakdown of AEA, you have more of the bliss molecule around for longer. It's a similar idea to the way most current antidepressant drugs work. Called selective serotonin reuptake inhibitors (SSRIs), they reduce the reuptake of serotonin after initial production, so there is more "left over" to continue signaling. This approach could be a viable alternative to actually giving people synthetic opioids like oxycodone and fentanyl that they easily become addicted to, instead allowing their natural opioids to persist longer for better control of mental and physical pain.

One natural approach to inhibiting FAAH and keeping AEA levels higher for longer is a related fatty acid molecule called palmitoylethanolamide (PEA). While PEA is not a traditional cannabinoid (because it does not actually bind to CB receptors), it can help to amplify the effects of the body's own endocannabinoids, especially AEA, by slowing the activity of FAAH and thus resulting in higher levels of the bliss molecule for longer. PEA is naturally found in egg yolks, soybeans, and peanuts, and nature-identical forms can be produced from a variety of vegetable oils as a source of fatty acids.

Immune System

Of all the signaling systems in our axis, our immune system is by far the most complex but also the most modifiable. In many ways, this makes it the most important target for our focus in improving vigor across mental and physical domains.

The gastrointestinal tract houses the densest concentration of immune cells in the body—with approximately 70 percent of our entire immune system residing in the gut. It is in constant contact with trillions of microbiome bacteria; with the nutrients, toxins, and pathogens from our diet; and with the intestinal lining that separates our "inside" (bloodstream) from the "outside" (the contents of our gut). This intestinal (visceral) layer is only a single cell thick, and a healthy gut lining is further protected by a thick layer of mucus, which is where most of the microbiome interactions occur. This dual lining of intestinal cells and mucus layer provides an environment for our gut to release small signaling molecules (cytokines/chemokines) to communicate with the immune system—and for the immune system to communicate with the rest of our body, including the HPA axis (stress response system), the heart, and the brain. Indeed, microbiome signaling can dramatically modulate immune system responses during infection, inflammation, stress, and autoimmunity.

For hundreds of years, most scientists considered the brain to be insulated from the immune system by the blood-brain barrier, but very recent research suggests that our immune system is intimately involved in brain function. The emerging scientific field of psychoneuroimmunology is completely revising the concept that our brain runs the body and the immune system protects it. Instead, we're conceiving of a much closer relationship, where the immune system closely regulates mood, mental function, and brain performance. New research shows how the immune system helps the brain cope with stress and supports essential brain functions such as learning and social interactions. In many ways, our immune system is much more than just a "shield" to protect us from bacterial and viral infections; it's more like a systemic body-wide surveillance organ. Similar to how our eyes send visual information and our ears send auditory information, our immune system detects and sends information about our internal and external environments to our brain.

The immune system has two major branches: innate immunity and adaptive immunity. Innate immunity initiates the inflammatory response, while adaptive immunity consists mainly of T and B lymphocytes that can recognize and attack specific pathogens. If the immune system becomes *underactive*—such as in response to chronic stress, sleep deprivation, burnout, or overtraining in athletes—this can lead to elevated risk for upper respiratory tract infections such as cold/flu and increased risk of cancer. If it becomes *overactive*, we might find excessive inflammation, allergies, and autoimmune conditions such as rheumatoid arthritis, multiple sclerosis, lupus, type 1 diabetes, and others. Innate immunity can be "primed," or brought back into balance, to help control inflammatory balance and enhance cancer vigilance through natural approaches, such as through the use of yeast and mushroom extracts.

The brain contains its own native immune cells called microglia, and the blood-brain barrier keeps peripheral innate and adaptive immune cells from entering the brain. Both the vagus nerve and cerebrospinal fluid can carry immune system signaling molecules (cytokines) into the brain, where they can help regulate many different brain functions. For example, cytokine signaling is thought to be involved in our response to chronic stress and may be the central disruption underlying related conditions, such as PTSD, fibromyalgia, and chronic fatigue syndrome.

In addition to cytokine signaling, the brain contains its own specialized type of waste-removal vessels to assist with cellular repair and toxin removal in place of immune system cleanup. Throughout the body, two types of vessels exist to move fluids to and from our tissues—much as your home's plumbing has separate water pipes and sewage pipes. Our blood vessels deliver oxygen and nutrients to our tissues, and our lymphatic vessels remove toxins and cellular waste products. The lymph vessels also contain lymph nodes that are enriched in immune cells to detect and address problems such as injury or infection in the tissues that they drain. The specialized lymphatic network that drains the brain (called the glymphatic system) includes a network of channels that circulate cerebrospinal fluid to both clean and detoxify the brain and circulate cytokines to provide information to the brain from the immune system—and vice versa. For example, one cytokine known as interleukin-1-beta (IL-1B) stimulates behaviors known as "sickness behavior" that many people exhibit when ill, such as excessive fatigue and sleep, decreased appetite, and social withdrawal. Other cytokines produced by the immune system, including interferon gamma and IL-17, can interact with neurons in the brain's prefrontal cortex to govern social behavior, including behaviors related to autism spectrum disorders. Because of the widespread ability of the innate immune system to recognize general patterns and types of bacterial/viral invaders and the adaptive immune system's ability for recognizing specific invaders, the immune system is increasingly being thought of by scientists as a "sense" in similar ways as smell, touch, taste, sight, and hearing. As a sixth sense, the immune system detects microorganisms and uses cytokines to inform the brain about them and modulate brain function and behavior.

Summary

Restoring balance across these multiple overlapping communication systems requires what an engineer might call a "systems approach" that entails a step-by-step analysis of what is going right or wrong at each stage of the communication process across the entire axis. This whole-body approach is exactly what we do within "functional medicine" and "functional nutrition" when we're trying to get to the root cause of a particular problem.

From the perspective of improving how we feel and perform across the entire mental wellness continuum, we can certainly "feel better" in a variety of ways by improving the function of any of our three brains (head, gut, or heart). However, by also restoring balance across our entire axis of communication between each brain and the rest of our body, we can realistically approach optimal levels of wellness across body and mind, achieving a state of mental fitness where we feel and perform at our peak potential.

The forthcoming chapters will outline many of the natural approaches that have been shown to be extremely effective in improving both mental and physical performance, including nutrition (and supplements), exercise, sleep, mindfulness, social connection, and many others.

PART 2

WHAT TO DO

In this part, we'll discuss some of the research-proven approaches to restoring microbiome balance, improving efficiency across the entire gut-heart-brain axis, and helping us achieve vigor in mind, body, and spirit.

Importantly, these approaches and tips are not just supported by scientific evidence but they're also doable. Science is great, but when that science can actually have a meaningful impact in your life in terms of how you feel and perform on a daily basis, then that is where it really gets exciting. As such, everything in part 2 has been specifically selected based on both the evidence for effectiveness and the likelihood for it to work in your actual life!

First, we will address the perennial question of what to eat. We'll outline the Mental Fitness Diet, which is not exactly a diet; it's an approach to food that has been shown to improve mood better than antidepressant drugs.

Next, we'll get you off your couch by outlining the importance (and joy) of whole-body movement, which is not exactly exercise. We'll also discuss how moving our body improves mental wellness better than prescription antianxiety drugs and sharpens our focus better than attention-deficit drugs.

It's a scary fact that our lack of sleep is not just putting us in a bad mood but it's also increasing our risk for cancer, diabetes, heart disease, and Alzheimer's disease. If that's not enough to keep you up at night, poor sleep quality makes us stressed, fat, less empathetic, and less in the mood for sex—none of which is good for our vigor. Surprisingly, while it might be difficult to actually get the eight hours of nightly sleep that most of us need, there are some very simple ways to improve sleep quality so that whatever amount of sleep you're able to get is more restorative for both mind and body.

It's important to address our social connections and the modern epidemic of disconnection. This discussion will help to restore our hope and self-efficacy in three areas: control (developing a sense that we can affect our fate), commitment (to a belief in the value of something that is important enough to work toward), and community (being an active part of a group that values the same things we do). Most of our struggles in life are less about "you versus someone else" and more about "you versus you" in a battle between our present and future selves.

Finally, we'll cover the dozens of natural supplements that can have a meaningful impact on our gut, brain, heart, and axis—with a specific emphasis on those that have both a long history of traditional use and solid scientific evidence for improving mental fitness.

This second part takes abstract scientific facts and distills them into a set of practical approaches you can apply to your busy life. As I often say, I love the science, but I love even more when we can apply the science to make a meaningful impact on our health and well-being—especially in how we feel and perform on a daily basis.

CHAPTER 5

THE MENTAL FITNESS DIET

Supporting your microbiome properly is like having a natural internal stress vaccine that activates automatically and on demand, whenever you need it. In dozens of studies, diet has been shown to be the most direct, immediate, and critical factor in maintaining a healthy microbiome as well as the health of the gut brain, the heart brain, and the head brain. As a result, diet is intimately linked with both mental wellness and physical health. Specific dietary interventions have been shown to be more effective than prescription antidepressant drugs in alleviating depression and antianxiety drugs in quelling anxiety, both in the initial effects to help you feel better quickly and in long-term prevention of future relapse.

Substantial changes in gut microbiome balance are measurable within as little as twenty-four hours following dietary change. For example, switching volunteers from a Western diet—one high in sugar, salt, and fat—to a diet higher in fiber-rich fruits and vegetables increases microbiome diversity and reduces systemic inflammation within forty-eight hours.

Perhaps the best-studied dietary format for improving both microbiome balance and psychological mood state is the Mediterranean diet, which consists mostly of whole grains, nuts, legumes, vegetables, and fruits, with moderate consumption of poultry and fish, and red meat consumed sparingly. Such dietary patterns result in distinctive improvements in gut microbiome balance and dramatically reduce the incidence of neuroinflammatory disorders such as Alzheimer's disease, psychiatric conditions such as depression, and cardiovascular conditions such as heart attack and stroke.

Individuals following a Mediterranean-style diet tend to consume higher levels of fiber (including prebiotic fibers), plant proteins, and phytonutrients (especially polyphenols, flavonoids, and carotenoids). Because of these plant-derived nutrients, people eating this way also display improved ratios of microbiome bacteria associated with enhanced metabolism and resistance to weight gain (higher Bacteroidetes and lower Firmicutes). Because amino acids are required building blocks for neurotransmitter synthesis, the high intake of plant proteins in a Mediterranean diet provides multifunctional benefits for mood (neurotransmitter synthesis), inflammatory balance (higher SCFA production), gut health (superior maintenance of gut mucosal barrier), and heart and brain health (lower systemic inflammation) compared to Western diets high in animal protein.

Diets high in animal fats, particularly saturated and trans fats, have been associated with elevated risk for not only psychological problems such as depression but also for cardiovascular disease, inflammatory gut diseases, and neurodegenerative diseases. High-fat diets have also been shown to adversely shift microbiome metabolism toward weight gain due to a decrease in Bacteroidetes and increase in Firmicutes levels. Conversely, omega-3 fatty acids found predominantly in fatty fish such as salmon, mackerel, sardine, and anchovies have been shown to increase "good" bacteria species, including *Bifidobacterium* and *Lactobacillus* levels. Likewise, the unique combination of plant proteins and prebiotic fibers (oligosaccharides) found in chickpeas (a staple of the Mediterranean diet) is known to shift the ratio of Firmicutes to Bacteroidetes downward toward one associated not just with fat loss but also with resistance to future weight gain.

Stressed Microbes

Our microbiome is also influenced by chemical exposure we may encounter through our diets and environment. The gut microbiome is known to metabolize—and be disrupted by—at least fifty environmental chemicals, including heavy metals and endocrine disruptors such as bisphenol A (BPA) found in many plastics. BPA in our food and environment has been shown to reduce gut microbiome diversity while increasing the ratios of "bad" bacteria associated with inflammation.

Perhaps the most detrimental "chemicals" that can induce widespread microbiome damage are antibiotics. Even if you have never *taken* an antibiotic medication (which is exceedingly rare), our *exposure* to them is almost constant because they contaminate our lakes, rivers, municipal water supplies (tap water), agricultural soil, and many food sources, particularly commercial sources of chicken, pork, and beef.

Even nonantibiotic drugs, whether taken directly or following exposure as environmental contaminants, have the potential to alter gut microbiome balance and influence mood and behavior. In addition to antibiotics, more than forty categories of drugs are known to adversely impact the microbiome, including laxatives (for constipation), proton pump inhibitors (for heartburn), female hormones (including birth control pills), metformin (for diabetes), statins (for cholesterol), IBD/IBS drugs (for gut problems), benzodiazepines (for anxiety), antihistamines (for allergies), and antidepressants.

With this long list of drugs that can damage our microbiome and the understanding that many individuals are subjected to a high degree of polypharmacy (taking multiple drugs for multiple conditions), it's little wonder that mental wellness issues are reaching epidemic proportions globally. As one particular example, the entire class of drugs most commonly prescribed to treat depression—the SSRIs including fluoxetine (Prozac), sertraline (Zoloft), paroxetine (Paxil), and others—are known to have antimicrobial activity, which results in a depletion of "good" bacteria, including *Lactobacillus, Prevotella, Akkermansia*, and others associated with metabolism and resistance to weight gain. This may explain a large part of the common side effect of weight gain in patients taking SSRIs.

Resilient Microbes

On a positive note, just as synthetic prescription antidepressant drugs are detrimental to the microbiome, dietary supplementation with probiotic bacteria, prebiotic fibers, and phytobiotic nutrients can be beneficial to microbiome diversity and resilience. A number of *Lactobacillus* and *Bifidobacterium* bacterial strains have been shown to reduce stress (including lower cortisol levels), anxiety (including higher GABA levels), and depression (including higher serotonin levels). Prebiotic fibers, particularly galacto-oligosaccharides (GOS) and galactomannan, have been shown to improve stress resilience, cognitive flexibility, and mental performance, likely through a combination of enhanced microbiome balance and reduced exposure to pro-inflammatory cytokines. Probiotics and prebiotics, and increasingly plant-extracted phytobiotics, are being shown to modulate microbiome balance and buffer the negative effects of both psychological and physical stress. For example, activation of the hypothalamic-pituitary-adrenal (HPA) axis stress response network is attenuated in response to exposure to both acute and chronic stressors, likely due to improvements in cortisol exposure, microbiome diversity, and gut integrity.

Dietary Patterns for Mental Fitness

I don't really like the term *diet* because it often implies a way of eating that you'll follow for a period of time and then stop. Most people think of a diet as a restrictive approach to eating that they'll eventually be "off" so they can go back to their "normal" way of eating.

A better term would be *habitual nutrition*. It actually just describes the kinds of foods that an animal or a person is typically eating on a regular or consistent basis. When viewed from this lens, it makes perfect sense to refer to the Mental Fitness Diet as a *pattern* of eating that you want to follow on a daily basis with as much meal-to-meal consistency as possible.

When we talk about diets, we need to always keep in mind that our meals are a diverse collection of nutrients that interact in a variety of ways to support our mental and physical health. So even though we can add a specific or isolated vitamin such as folate (vitamin B9), a mineral like magnesium, or a fatty acid like omega-3s to support mental fitness, we need to keep the "whole diet" in mind at all times.

You'll see in the sections to follow that one of the primary approaches underlying the entire Mental Fitness Diet is simply to eat more plants, especially more brightly colored, high-fiber fruits and vegetables. Writer Michael Pollan had it exactly right when he summed it all up with seven words in his excellent book *Food Rules* as "eat food, not too much, mostly plants." He further defines *food* as "real food," such as whole vegetables, fruits, whole grains, and fish, as opposed to "edible food-like substances" (by which he means processed junk food).

One look at the Mental Fitness Diet Food Pyramid (see next page) reveals that at least *half* of your plate should be covered by vegetables, fruits, and spices (the "base" of the pyramid). The other half of your plate is a balanced combination of whole grains, beans/legumes/seeds/nuts, and healthy proteins/fats (which always come in combination). This "plant slant" does not mean that meat is bad, but rather it helps to focus us on the fact that plant foods contain a vast array of the specific bioactive compounds that help us feel better now and remain feeling great in the future, especially when we're under stress (boosting our resilience).

Without getting too much into the botany and biochemistry of plants, many of the healthiest plant compounds—such as flavonoids, carotenoids, glucosinolates, and many others—are produced by the plant to provide natural stress protection against the damaging effects of sunlight, heat, drought, and pests. When we ingest the plants in our diets, we get those anti-stress benefits as well! In our own human bodies, these anti-stress plant compounds help support microbiome balance, reduce cellular damage (antioxidant effects), restore immune vigilance (and cancer surveillance), balance inflammation (for heart and brain health), boost blood flow (supporting both mental and physical performance), and help with hormonal balance and blood sugar control.

MENTAL WELLNESS FOOD PYRAMID

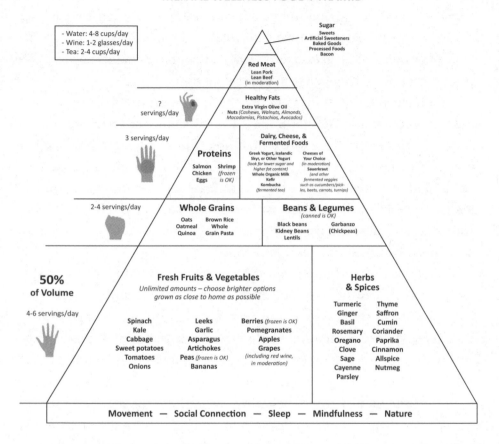

- Water: 4-8 cups/day
- Wine: 1-2 glasses/day
- Tea: 2-4 cups/day

Sugar
Sweets
Artificial Sweeteners
Baked Goods
Processed Foods
Bacon

Red Meat
Lean Pork
Lean Beef
(in moderation)

?
servings/day

Healthy Fats
Extra Virgin Olive Oil
Nuts *(Cashews, Walnuts, Almonds, Macadamias, Pistachios, Avocados)*

3 servings/day

Proteins
Salmon   Shrimp
Chicken   *(frozen*
Eggs   *is OK)*

Dairy, Cheese, & Fermented Foods
Greek Yogurt, Icelandic   Cheeses of
Skyr, or Other Yogurt   Your Choice
(look for lower sugar and   *(in moderation)*
higher fat content)   Sauerkraut
Whole Organic Milk   *(and other*
Kefir   *fermented veggies*
Kombucha   *such as cucumbers/pick-*
(fermented tea)   *les, beets, carrots, turnips)*

2-4 servings/day

Whole Grains
Oats   Brown Rice
Oatmeal   Whole
Quinoa   Grain Pasta

Beans & Legumes
(canned is OK)
Black beans   Garbanzo
Kidney Beans   (Chickpeas)
Lentils

50%
of Volume

4-6 servings/day

Fresh Fruits & Vegetables
Unlimited amounts – choose brighter options grown as close to home as possible

Spinach   Leeks   Berries *(frozen is OK)*
Kale   Garlic   Pomegranates
Cabbage   Asparagus   Apples
Sweet potatoes Artichokes   Grapes
Tomatoes   Peas *(frozen is OK)* *(including red wine,*
Onions   Bananas   *in moderation)*

Herbs & Spices
Turmeric   Thyme
Ginger   Saffron
Basil   Cumin
Rosemary   Coriander
Oregano   Paprika
Clove   Cinnamon
Sage   Allspice
Cayenne   Nutmeg
Parsley

Movement — Social Connection — Sleep — Mindfulness — Nature

Plant foods are rich in all of the standard essential nutrients such as vitamins, minerals, fatty acids, carbohydrates, protein, and fiber, but they are also packed with thousands of bioactive phytonutrients such as flavonoids (found in berries, grapes, apples, citrus, tea, red wine, and dark chocolate), carotenoids (found in carrots, peppers, squash, sweet potatoes, spinach, and kale), thiols/glucosinolates (found in onions, garlic, leeks, brussels sprouts, broccoli, and cabbage), and lignans/phytoestrogens (found in nuts, seeds, beans, whole grains, and chickpeas). As such, plants form the base of the Mental Fitness Diet pyramid and—I cannot emphasize this enough—should represent *at least half* of the food on your plate at each meal.

Research studies around the world have repeatedly shown that people who follow a Mediterranean-style diet with lots of plants and seafood have about a 50 percent reduction in their risk for developing depression compared to people who eat more of a Western-style dietary pattern filled with fast and processed food, such as refined grains. In other studies, a traditional Japanese dietary pattern rich in fish, green tea, green leafy vegetables, tofu, and fermented foods has been associated with half as much depression and half as many suicides as Japanese eating more of a Western-style diet. The very same dramatic reductions in mental wellness issues have been shown across Scandinavia (Norway, Finland, Sweden, Denmark, and Iceland) among people eating more of a traditional whole-foods dietary pattern compared to a Western-style diet higher in red meat, refined grains, and processed foods. Diet is clearly a dominant factor underlying the reason that these countries are routinely atop the global lists of "happiest places" around the world. It's also interesting that numerous studies have shown that countries with the highest consumption of seafood (especially fatty fish) have dramatically lower rates of mental disorders such as anxiety, ADHD, and depression (including postpartum/postnatal depression).

Again and again, we are repeatedly seeing the same pattern emerge from research studies around the world in more and more countries—that higher dietary intake of less-processed, whole foods will improve mood, while higher intakes of processed foods will reduce mood. This relationship is observed in men and women—younger and older, leaner and fatter, richer and poorer, active and sedentary—and across the animal kingdom, including mice, rats, and chimpanzees. In the animal studies, researchers have shown not only changes in behavior (like depression, anxiety, social isolation, and more) but also changes in neurotransmitters such as serotonin (happy neurotransmitter) and GABA (relaxation neurotransmitter) as well as direct changes in microbiome balance and brain structure. In the brain, junk food diets reduce the growth of new neurons, especially in the hippocampus, an area of the brain important for not just mental health but also learning and memory.

It's important to note that the effects of dietary patterns on mood and mental performance seem to be independent of each other—meaning that eating more healthy foods does not "cancel out" eating a lot of unhealthy junk foods. Likewise, avoiding junk food and processed food but also avoiding vegetables, fruits, and whole grains is also problematic for mental fitness.

One of the very interesting biological responses to processed foods is that they tend to activate the body's internal stress response systems (including the adrenal glands, microbiome, and immune system). And vice versa, an overactive or chronic stress response often leads to "stress-eating" and cravings for more junk food—setting off a vicious cycle of stress followed by stress-eating followed by a continued stress response.

Not only is following a Mental Fitness Diet good for your mood and mental performance, it's also effective in preventing dementia, heart disease, and diabetes. Several studies have shown that eating a Mental Fitness Diet pattern (high in vegetables, fruits, beans, nuts, whole grains, fish, olive oil; moderate in red wine; and low in red meat and dairy) reduces rates of cognitive decline, dementia, and Alzheimer's disease, including direct reductions in the accumulation of amyloid proteins. The world's largest diet intervention study, the PREDIMED trial (Prevención con Dieta Mediterránea) followed more than seven thousand European adults between the ages of fifty-five to eighty with high risk factors for heart disease. The volunteers followed a Mediterranean-style diet (very similar to the Mental Fitness Diet) or a low-fat diet recommended by the American Heart Association. The study was designed to run for six years but was stopped after only five years when it became clear that people on the Mediterranean diet already had a substantial 30 percent reduction in heart attacks compared to the low-fat diet. They also had better cognitive function, less diabetes, lower blood pressure, lower cholesterol, and reductions in measures of oxidative stress and inflammation.

In another very large study (the Harvard Nurses' Health Study) that tracked habitual diet patterns over time in forty-five thousand women—versus actually altering diets like PREDIMED—those who ate closer to a

Mental Fitness Diet pattern had approximately 40 percent lower inflammation than those who adhered closer to a Western diet pattern. This is an important finding because of the close links between inflammation, immune function, and depression.

One of the more groundbreaking studies linking dietary patterns to mental fitness was the SMILES (Supporting the Modification of lifestyle in Lowered Emotional States) trial in Australia. Depressed subjects in this trial followed a Mediterranean-style diet for twelve weeks, with a complete remission of depressive symptoms in a third of participants. A similar twelve-week Australian study (HELFIMED, which stands for Healthy Eating for Life with a Mediterranean-style diet) showed a prevention of developing depression in the first place. Taken together, these intervention studies (where volunteers follow a dietary pattern and report back over time) provide convincing evidence that a Mediterranean-style diet, which is similar to the Mental Fitness Diet, can both treat depression in those who have it and prevent it in people at risk for it.

In a more recent intervention study (Project b3—Brain, Body, Biome), my research group has shown that the Mental Fitness Diet can even help "healthy stressed" people. While these folks might not be diagnosed with depression or anxiety disorders, they certainly have a degree of stress in their lives, don't eat a perfect diet, don't get eight hours of nightly sleep, and don't exercise as much as they know they should. Does that sound like anyone you know? Our subjects experienced dramatic improvements of 30 to 60 percent in overall mood, energy, focus, and resilience (more about this study and how you can apply it to your own life in the final chapter).

Building Buff Brains

At this point, we know that dietary patterns defined by high-sugar processed foods and low in fiber-rich, phytonutrient-filled whole foods are bad for our mood, focus, and overall mental fitness. We also know that processed foods are viewed as a "threat" by our microbiome (second brain), setting off a stress response (adrenals/cortisol) that includes an immune activation and an inflammatory reaction ("axis") that can damage our heart (third brain) and destroy neurons (first brain). This response to a Western diet is almost exactly like what happens when we encounter a bacterial or viral infection—the body leaps into action across multiple systems to "protect" us from the threatening invader. Unfortunately, when we're "dosing" ourselves multiple times every day with junk food poisons, our axis systems become reprogrammed to be in a state of constant overactivity—leading to a chronic overload of cortisol, inflammatory cytokines, and tissue breakdown.

Consuming more of a Mental Fitness Diet not only reduces the damage across our entire gut-heart-brain axis but actually encourages the growth of new neurons in many areas of the brain. Numerous studies, including some of my own, have recently shown that eating styles similar to the Mental Fitness Diet increase levels of a protein growth factor known as brain-derived neurotrophic factor (BDNF)—even in middle-aged and older adults. BDNF packs a dual benefit because it can both protect existing brain neurons from oxidative and inflammatory stress and promote the growth of new neurons in key brain regions (like the hippocampus) associated with memory, emotions, mood, and mental fitness. People with depression and bipolar disorder often have reduced hippocampal volume and lower levels of BDNF.

We've known for some time that stress reduces BDNF, while exercise elevates it. Now we have another tool—our diet—to help protect and actually *build* our brain. Think about how much effort some people (myself included) put into exercising and eating right to build a healthy, strong, high-performance body; the exact same principles apply for building a healthy, strong, high-performance brain.

Your Mental Fitness Diet Journey

Please give me two weeks, and I'll help you understand not just what to eat but why you're eating it and how the heck you can easily prepare this weird food (kale!?) that you might not even recognize the first time you look for it in the produce department of your local grocery store.

We're going to take baby steps—one step per day for the next fourteen days. You'll start feeling better on the very first day, and you'll feel better and better each day until you feel amazing by the end of the two weeks. You'll also be set up for feeling great for the rest of your life if you continue implementing the simple steps that we'll focus on in the next section. Don't worry—we're not setting off to make you into a professional chef. Instead, we're looking for ways to insert the biggest bang (mental fitness boost) for the smallest buck (your time and effort) so you reap the greatest rewards within your already busy life.

The Mental Fitness Diet is, at its essence, simply a framework to help you eat less processed junk food and more whole food. All the research summarized earlier comes down to a very simple fact: if you eat crap, you feel like crap. But the converse is also true—and supported by research— that if you eat more whole food, you will feel more whole in body and mind and you'll reap significant improvements in both physical and mental fitness.

Don't be scared. It's a lot easier—and tastier—than you might think.

In the following section, I give you a short highlight of the concept or principle that the particular day is intended to cover. But, because each of these tips is most effective when you can actually integrate them into your busy life, I strongly believe that seeing them come to life (in a video) can really help underscore the principles you're reading about here. As such, the Mental Fitness TV website has a series of free videos to guide you through each day and every recipe. I strongly encourage you to visit MentalFitness.tv to see how you can turn these ideas into actions.

DAY 1 WHAT NOT TO EAT (THE "STOP EATING CRAP" PLAN)

This is the "intervention" portion of our plan—the things we need to *stop* doing before we can move along to the things that we can *start* doing with our eating behaviors. The research is quite clear on the fact that eating more of the "good stuff" (fiber, phytonutrients, fermented foods, healthy fats, and plant-based proteins) can help us feel better, but the research is equally clear on the contrary fact that eating crap leads us very quickly to feeling like crap. Sorry to be so blunt, but somebody has to say it.

The Mental Fitness Diet is not just about adding more of the good stuff; it's also about getting rid of *some* of the bad stuff. These actions work independently of each other to push your mood up or down. Even if you're adding a lot of the good, it won't really "make up for" a continued intake of the bad. To be clear, this is not to say that we can never indulge in a chocolate chip cookie or a piece of cake, but we need to be more mindful of how often we do that.

As described earlier, this style or *pattern* of eating has been shown in multiple clinical trials to be more effective than prescription antidepressants in improving mood and reducing depression. The combination of fiber, healthy fat, fermented foods, phytonutrients (what we refer to as "good mood foods"), and the lower intake of sugar and processed foods combine to improve microbiome balance, gut health, and overall gut-brain axis balance.

DAY 2 FRESH FRUITS AND VEGETABLES

Fresh fruits and vegetables are medicine—pure and simple. Besides the high fiber content, which nourishes our good bacteria, fruits and vegetables are rich sources of antioxidants that can protect our health at the cellular level.

DAY 3 WHOLE GRAINS AND LEGUMES

Whole grains, legumes, seeds, nuts, and beans seem tailor-made to support our entire gut-heart-brain axis. Because these are rich sources of phytonutrients, fiber, and healthy fats, each of these superfoods can also help to modulate blood sugar levels (which supports overall metabolism and mental performance) while simultaneously improving gut health and supporting gut integrity.

DAY 4 PROTEINS AND DAIRY

Protein is vital to building and repairing every tissue in our body, including muscles, tendons, ligaments, bones, skin, and every one of our ten trillion body cells. As we age, we may require more protein to maintain energy levels and muscle strength. Likewise, if we're trying to lose body fat or gain muscle, we need an even higher daily intake of protein. Incorporating lean protein sources—balanced with fruits/vegetables and healthy fats—can actually help us "age better," adding more life to our years. For nonmeat options, consider beans, seeds, nuts, and plant-based proteins such as chickpeas.

DAY 5 HEALTHY FATS

Fat is not your enemy! Healthy fats like those found in fish, olives, avocados, seeds, and nuts are a vital building block for healthy brain cells. Healthy fats help to modulate overall metabolism, so eating the *right* fat can actually help you *burn more* fat! Fat also helps our foods taste good— and helps to improve satiety, so we feel fuller for longer.

DAY 6 RED MEAT

Red meat may no longer be the center of attention, and it sure as heck should not be the main focus of any meal, but that doesn't mean it has to be eliminated completely. Red meat represents the richest source of protein available, so it can definitely be an important part of a healthy, well-balanced Mental Fitness Diet. But since overconsumption is clearly shown to increase systemic inflammation (across our gut-heart-head brains), we need to consume red meat in moderation to modulate inflammation within a healthy range. Red meat still holds a healthy place in your diet, but more as a condiment or a side dish than as a main course.

DAY 7   A Healthy Sweet Tooth

It's no secret that sweets and processed foods aren't recommended for healthy eating of any kind, let alone for mental fitness. But remember that mental fitness is about feeling our best and about enjoying all aspects of life—and indulging in a sweet treat now and then is one of life's great joys. There are numerous ways for us to enjoy a little sweetness without going overboard.

DAY 8   Making It Work for You

Now that you know the Mental Fitness Diet, let's learn how to make it work for you with shopping lists, meal plans, and tips and tricks for preparing for the week.

DAY 9   Meal Prepping and Smoothie Packs

You've heard of meal prepping, but now we'll tackle how it can save you time and energy while implementing the Mental Fitness Diet.

DAY 10   Healthy Eating with Kids (or Picky Adults)

Do you have kids? Then you probably want them to eat better. Let's show you how.

DAY 11   No Cooking Required

Let's start with the easiest form of cooking—NONE! Learn how to make quick and easy meals that require no cooking.

DAY 12   Sheet pan Cooking

Sheet pan cooking is all the rage. Learn how it works perfectly with this eating plan.

DAY 13   SKILLET MEALS

Need to cook something fast? Learn how to do it in a skillet. You + a Pan + a Plan = an easy and delicious mental fitness meal.

DAY 14   KEEP GOING & EASY ONE-POT MEALS

Wrap up the journey with one last awesome meal that takes advantage of the hottest new trend: one-pot or "Instant Pot" meals.

Summary

That doesn't sound too bad, does it?

Now you've seen what the fourteen-day plan looks like. Does it feel doable?

If you stick with it for two weeks and then keep eating this way on a regular basis (a.k.a. your new "diet"), you'll notice that you feel better (stress, energy, tension) and better (memory, focus, creativity) and better (mood, resilience, vigor) over time.

Read on for the details about diving into your new way of eating.

Mental Fitness Diet Shopping List

It's a good idea to have as many of these items on hand as possible so you're always prepared to whip something healthy together, preventing the urge to eat processed junk.

Fresh Fruits and Vegetables

➤ Unlimited amounts—choose brighter options grown as close to home as possible

➤ Spinach

➤ Kale

➤ Cabbage

➤ Sweet potatoes

➤ Squash

- Tomatoes
- Peppers (the more colors the better—red, orange, yellow, green, and hot!)
- Onions
- Leeks
- Garlic
- Broccoli (frozen is OK)
- Cauliflower (frozen is OK)
- Fennel
- Asparagus
- Artichokes

Beans and Legumes

- Canned is OK
- Black beans
- Kidney beans

Healthy Fats

- Extra-virgin olive oil
- Avocados
- Nuts—cashews, walnuts,

Whole Grains

- Oats/oatmeal
- Whole grain pasta

- Peas (frozen is OK)
- Green beans
- Bananas and plantains
- Berries—blueberries, blackberries, raspberries (frozen is OK)
- Pomegranates
- Apples
- Citrus fruits (oranges, tangerines, lemons, limes, grapefruit)
- Grapes (including red wine, in moderation)

- Garbanzos (chickpeas)
- Lentils

almonds, macadamias, pistachios

- Quinoa
- Brown rice

Dairy, Cheese, and Fermented Foods

➤ Greek yogurt, Icelandic Skyr, or other yogurt (look for lower sugar and higher fat content)

➤ Whole organic milk

➤ Kefir

➤ Kombucha (fermented tea)

➤ Cheeses of your choice (in moderation)

➤ Sauerkraut

➤ Other fermented veggies (such as cucumbers/pickles, beets, carrots, turnips)

Proteins

➤ Salmon

➤ Tuna (canned is OK)

➤ Chicken (fresh or frozen)

➤ Eggs

➤ Shrimp (frozen is OK)

➤ Lean pork

➤ Lean beef (in moderation)

➤ Seitan (a vegan meat substitute made from wheat gluten)

➤ Tofu, tempeh, and edamame (all different versions of soy)

Herbs and Spices

➤ Turmeric

➤ Ginger

➤ Basil

➤ Rosemary

➤ Oregano

➤ Clove

➤ Sage

➤ Cayenne

➤ Parsley

➤ Thyme

➤ Saffron

➤ Cumin

➤ Coriander

➤ Paprika

➤ Cinnamon

➤ Allspice

➤ Nutmeg

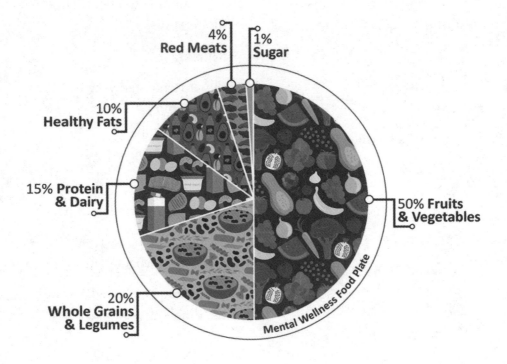

4% **Red Meats**

1% **Sugar**

10% **Healthy Fats**

15% **Protein & Dairy**

50% **Fruits & Vegetables**

20% **Whole Grains & Legumes**

Mental Wellness Food Plate

CHAPTER 6

MOVEMENT FOR MENTAL FITNESS

I'm a bit of an exercise nut. I was a very mediocre athlete in high school, where I was part of the track team—less as a competitive athlete and more for the social aspect. In college, a friend encouraged me to give rowing (crew) a try. I was instantly hooked! Crew ended up becoming an aspect of my college life on par in importance (or even more so) with my studies in sports medicine and fitness management. The actual on-water rowing was intense enough, but add in the rowing machines, running, and weight lifting workouts, and we were exercising for a couple of hours every day. After my rowing career, I took up bicycle racing and then triathlons and eventually ultramarathons. At this point, I've completed several dozen Ironman distance triathlons and fifty- to one-hundred-mile off-road ultras. You might even say that I'm now "addicted" to exercise, or at least reliant on exercise in certain ways—especially to maintain my mental fitness.

I often ask my students who exercise whether or not they would still do it if a study came out proving that exercise is "bad" for your health. The vast majority say that they would still exercise for the mental benefits and how exercise makes them feel. This can sound crazy to people who are not regular exercisers, because the perception of exercise is often one of being out of breath, sweaty, and uncomfortable—the familiar "no pain, no gain" message that many associate with exercise being a chore or a punishment.

I get it. Motivating yourself to exercise can be difficult when there are so many other enticing options to keep us sedentary, like soft couches, interesting television, and exciting video games. The list is endless. But I want to make the case in this chapter that regular physical movement—whether we call that exercise or not—is as vital for optimal mental fitness as nutrition, microbiome balance, or anything else covered in this book.

In many ways, my use of the word *diet* in the Mental Fitness Diet—which refers not to restriction but to "habitual consumption" of and "habitual exposure" to foods and nutrients—also applies to physical activity (what your *body* is routinely exposed to or doing) and to mindfulness practices (what your *mind* is routinely exposed to or thinking about). If we routinely expose our body to the right levels of physical movement, we can maintain balance across our entire gut-heart-brain axis and, in doing so, optimize both physical performance and mental performance.

The human body is a very unique type of "machine" that breaks down from both "overuse" (like all machines) as well as from "underuse" or being sedentary (unique to the human machine). The phrase "use it or lose it" is undoubtedly true for the human machine, and this chapter will help explain why movement is vital for mental fitness.

Movement as a Brain Builder

Moderate amounts of exercise can make a meaningful difference to brain function (including neurogenesis), heart function (including heart strength and efficiency), and gut function (including gut barrier function and microbiome diversity).

Older adults who can cover at least four hundred yards (about a quarter mile) in a standard six-minute walk test have half the risk of dying in the subsequent decade than their peers who can't make it three hundred yards, proving the "longevity" benefits of physical fitness. However, exercise does a lot more than just strengthen our hearts, bones, and muscles; it also reduces chronic inflammation, balances hormone levels, and blunts our physiologic response to stress—all of which are beneficial for mental fitness. Chronic inflammation and stress are indiscriminate killers, increasing our risk for heart disease, cancer, diabetes, neurological disease, and mental health problems.

Our brain starts to shrink around the age of forty, with cells deteriorating most quickly in the frontal lobe, the striatum, and the hippocampus—areas involved in our most complex thoughts, movement, and memory. How resistant you are to the effects of this decline is likely to be associated with your "cognitive reserve," a type of "mental buffer" that allows your brain to sustain more damage before you notice changes in your cognition, mood, or behavior. A great deal of cognitive reserve is related not necessarily to the sheer number of neurons you have but to how well those neurons engage with one another across different networks in the brain. The connection efficiency of our neurons is what enables our brain to compensate when age-related decline starts to occur, and it also helps reroute information so the organ can continue to operate optimally.

We know that inflammation, insulin resistance, stress, sleep loss, and social isolation will reduce cognitive reserve, while proper diet, education, adequate sleep, social connection, and exercise can boost it (even into our nineties). The old adage of "healthy body, healthy mind" has never been more true, with numerous research studies showing how regular physical activity yields dramatic improvements in memory, attention, processing speed, and executive functions such as planning and multitasking.

Exercise keeps our body fit, but it also improves brain fitness by increasing blood flow to the brain and stimulating the release of molecules that both stimulate the generation of new brain cells and keep older ones healthy. Physical movement also challenges the brain to coordinate myriad signals involved in balance, posture, and navigation, helping to maintain (and improve) our cognitive reserve and ward off dementia.

Counterintuitively, one thing that exercise doesn't do very well is increase our daily energy expenditure. Recent research has shown that total daily calorie burn is about the same between members of African hunter-gatherer cultures (Hadza tribe) and typical American adults—despite the Hadza being five to ten times more active. The difference comes down to the Hadza having adjusted their physically active lifestyle by spending less energy on other tasks—being strategically lazy—so total daily calorie expenditure remains constant. Being physically active does not seem to change the total number of calories your body spends each day but rather how you spend them.

The Hadza tribe are well studied for their unique microbiome, which is much more diverse and resilient compared to a typical Western microbiome. This is due in large part to their massive fiber intake (around 100 to 150 grams daily compared to a typical American intake of 10 to 15 grams and a recommended target of 30 to 40 grams per day) and also to their activity levels. A typical day in the life of a Hadza hunter-gatherer involves at least two hours of vigorous activity (such as running) and several hours of light activity (like walking). Compare that to the average sedentary American who is moving only about ten minutes per day. As a result of the vast differences in physical activity levels (and subsequent superior microbiome balance, which is partly due to fiber intake and partly due to movement), the Hadza have a better gut brain and show virtually no signs of cardiovascular disease (heart brain) or depression/anxiety (head brain).

In our typically sedentary lives, the body has an overabundance of readily available calories. As a result, physiological activities such as inflammation and the fight-or-flight stress response, which are normally short-lived and sporadic (acute), are abnormally "always on," raging in the background (chronic).

The latest research suggests that the optimum amount of daily exercise for mental and physical health and overall longevity is around fifteen thousand steps at vigorous intensity. This is roughly equivalent to about two hours per day of brisk walking—which might seem like far too much for the average modern busy lifestyle to accommodate. Luckily, lower durations of exercise undertaken at a somewhat higher intensity have also been shown to deliver dramatic body and mind benefits. For example, one eight-year study showed that twenty-five minutes of moderate-to-vigorous activity daily reduced the risk of dying by 25 percent. But more is even better. Those who were active for one hundred minutes per day had death rates 80 percent lower than their couch potato counterparts.

A recent Australian study of 150,000 adults showed that about an hour per day of vigorous activity is needed to counteract the detrimental health effects of sitting during work hours (as many of us do at our desks or behind a computer). A number of exercise scientists, including myself, are beginning to think of sitting as the "new smoking." We're learning that sitting for long periods—even if you're a regular exerciser—is shockingly bad for our overall physical and mental fitness. The more hours that you stay seated in a given day, the higher your risk for heart disease, diabetes, and cancer. It makes sense that we want to sit less, but we can also sit better with a couple of little adjustments.

Consider our hunter-gatherer friends, the Hadza. They are notorious "non-sitters" because of their near-constant level of movement through-out the day. But they also spend about nine hours per day sitting! Impor-tantly, they don't sit the way you or I do—by plopping down on a couch or an office chair—but rather by squatting or sitting on the ground in various positions. Studies using activity monitors have shown that even when sitting, the Hadza have significant levels of muscle activity because they are never in a single static position for very long. We can replicate this pattern with our own approach to more active sitting by frequently getting up or changing positions (for example, standing up from your office chair at least every hour), by using a higher stool to lean against or a kneeling chair, by sitting on a balance ball, or even by getting a standing desk. Any of these—or using all of them intermittently throughout the day (as I do)—can make a meaningful difference in the toll that sitting can take on our physical and mental fitness.

When looked at as a whole, the physical activity research broadly indicates that the most dangerous "dosage" of exercise is "none" and that any amount above that is beneficial (up to a point). For most people, a daily target of thirty minutes of daily heart-rate-elevating activity (enough where you're somewhat short of breath) would halve mortality rate—and would additionally help us feel better so we come back for more.

Movement as a Mood Modulator

Over generations of evolutionary development, our brain evolved to reward regular physical activity, releasing endorphins to inhibit pain and endocannabinoids to elevate mood. However, research also shows us that you don't have to be a fitness nut to reap the mental benefits from exercise. I like to refer to people who move their bodies regularly as "actives" instead of as "exercisers," to remove some of the negative connotations associated with exercise being a chore. All over the globe, research studies have shown that physically active people are happier and have higher life-satisfaction scores than their sedentary counterparts. Interestingly, these measures of overall well-being and higher quality of life have little to do with being "in shape," per se, and have more to do with simply the act of moving our bodies on a daily basis. No matter the type or intensity of activity (walking, running, biking, weights, yoga, organized sports, whatever), those "actives" who do anything are less likely to suffer from depression, anxiety, or loneliness (even if they are solo exercisers). Actives also tend to have a much higher sense of gratitude and stronger sense of purpose as well as a tendency toward hope and love, especially in times of stress. Actives tend to be "happier" than non-actives, but why?

There seem to be a number of contributing factors to the feel-good effects of being physically active. Partly it's the increase in neurotransmitters like endorphins and endocannabinoids—which is perhaps one of the reasons physical activity is superior to prescription drugs for alleviating depression and anxiety. Partly it's that the muscles themselves can gobble up stress hormones like cortisol and secrete other hormones like oxytocin (often called the "cuddle" hormone or the "connection" hormone) that enable us to engage with and connect with others. Partly it's that activity also results in lower levels of inflammatory markers, improves microbiome diversity, enhances gut motility, and actually stimulates brain plasticity (growth and rewiring of the brain to enhance not just cognition and memory but also receptivity to happiness and social connection and resilience to stress). If you had a prescription drug that could deliver even a fraction of these benefits, it would be the biggest blockbuster medicine of all time.

Evolutionary biologists have described physical movement as being essential to the entire human experience and the core of what it actually means to be human. Why else would our biology have so many ways to "reward" being active? The more we move, the better we feel, the clearer we think, the more connected and hopeful we become, and the longer we live with abundant health. Sounds like the very definition of a positive cycle! Unfortunately, the cycle spins the other way as well, with numerous research studies showing that while people are clearly happier on days when they are more physically active, periods of inactivity lead to higher levels of stress, fatigue, anxiety, and depression.

Activity as a Drug

So you feel better when you're "doing" it, and you have a noticeable "comedown" when you're "off" of it? Sounds like an addictive drug, right? We're not talking about caffeine, nicotine, alcohol, or any of the really addictive drugs like cocaine, heroin, or opiates—just exercise. We talked about the human microbiome as a natural "internal pharmacy," producing neurotransmitters on demand when we need them for happiness, motivation, focus, relaxation, and more. Likewise, the same on-demand production of natural internal neurochemicals and signaling molecules can be undertaken by our head brain and our heart brain, and even by our muscles.

You've probably heard of the "runner's high," that feeling of euphoria that accompanies a hard workout. You've probably also heard that this feeling is due to compounds called endorphins produced during exercise. We certainly produce endorphins during exercise, particularly during vigorous or intense exercise, but recent research indicates that endorphins are related more to suppression of pain sensations than they are to elevated mood. A different set of neurochemicals called endocannabinoids is responsible for the feel-good effects of physical activity, and research shows that we maximally produce both endorphins and endocannabi-noids when exercise intensity is moderate and sustained—or about the same speed we might associate with jogging for an hour or so after some wild game. The endorphins are reducing our pain and sending a "don't stop" signal to our muscles while the endocannabinoids are boosting our mood and sending a "keep going" signal to our brain. These subtly different signals combine to keep us persistently moving toward our goal—brilliant!

We know that even very light activity, such as walking, can help us feel better, but these effects are due to factors other than endorphins and endocannabinoids. For example, walking your dog stimulates blood flow to all parts of your body, including your head brain and heart brain; exposes you to nature and sunlight; and gently stimulates gut-brain motil-ity—all of which can help balance neurotransmitters such as serotonin and lead us to feel generally better. Production of endorphins and endo-cannabinoids need a little more oomph to get them going, with a sustained moderate effort that gets your heart rate and breathing rate elevated for twenty to thirty minutes. The combined effect of these activity-generated compounds is a general sense of contentment, which can reduce anxiety, lessen stress, and fuel optimism. Indeed, we know from (bad) experience that blocking these endocannabinoid signals can lead to profound spikes in depression, anxiety, and suicidal ideation. The weight loss drug Rimon-abant was approved in Europe in 2006 for its effects on blocking endo-cannabinoid receptors to suppress appetite, but it was removed from the market in 2009 and never approved in the USA because of the extreme psychological disturbances that it induced, including suicide.

Endocannabinoid receptors have been found throughout all parts of the body, but they are particularly concentrated across the gut-heart-brain axis. In the head brain, especially in the amygdala (fear center) and prefrontal cortex (creativity center), endocannabinoids can help induce calmness and engagement. In the heart brain, endocannabinoids can help to smooth electrical rhythms and stimulate oxytocin synthesis, both of which can help foster social connectedness. In the gut brain, endocannabinoid receptors are particularly enriched, especially in areas associated with immune vigilance such as the Peyer's patches and lymphoid tissues (which are also an important portion of the "axis"). This brings in another part of the endocannabinoid equation, with one side being the production of endocannabinoids that "activate" cellular receptors and the other side being the receptors themselves that "receive" those signals. The activation signal comes from the endocannabinoid compound, so we can generate more signals with physical activity or by supplementing plant versions (phytocannabinoids from hemp, vanilla, hot peppers, and more), but it needs to be received by the receptor. We can also increase the number and sensitivity of our receptors, with both physical activity and another class of phytonutrients called polyphenols (found in berries, apples, grapes, citrus, and many other foods). Activity is a one-two punch that delivers both the endocannabinoid signal and enhances the body's cellular response to those signals at the receptor level. This is one of the reasons exercise might feel difficult at first but gets more and more enjoyable the more you do it and eventually can become something that you "need" to do on a daily basis (as it is for me).

Endocannabinoids certainly have their own direct effects in many areas that help improve our mental fitness, but they also seem to have a cascade of indirect effects that improve our motivation (dopamine in the head brain), social connection (oxytocin in the heart brain), and relaxation (GABA in the gut brain). That combination of emotion-signaling molecules is what leads to sensations of not just feeling better but also of trust, belonging, and bonding. It's why athletes who compete on the same team, soldiers who fight in the same troop, and even married couples who work out together all develop stronger connections.

Another class of natural signaling molecules in the body is known as myokines. These are similar to the cytokines outlined in earlier chapters involved in cell-to-cell signaling and immune system regulation, but they emanate from our muscles (*myo* means "muscle," and *kine* means "movement"). When we move, our muscles secrete a wide range of myokines that signal the rest of our body to regulate metabolism, burn fat, control inflammation, prime the immune system, and balance stress and mood. One myokine in particular—named irisin after the Greek messenger goddess Iris—serves as a master signaling molecule and has been dubbed by many researchers as the "exercise hormone" for its ability to signal many of the beneficial effects of exercise, especially fat loss ("browning" of adipose tissue), antiaging (shortening of telomeres), and mental fitness (stimulation of neurogenesis). Another muscle-derived protein called PGC (short for peroxisome proliferator-activated receptor-gamma coactivator 1-alpha) has been called the "hope molecule" because it can directly influence mood, stress resilience, and mental fitness. The combined effects of irisin and PGC have been shown to promote fat loss and muscle gain, optimize metabolism of fat and glucose, and stimulate growth of neurons in the hippocampus region of the brain (associated with cognition and memory).

Clinical studies conducted all around the globe have shown repeatedly that exercise is not just effective for improving mood, but it is actually much *more* effective than prescription medications in alleviating both depression and anxiety. Compared to drugs, exercise has superior mood-boosting effects initially (getting patients from depressed to nondepressed) as well as over time (keeping people from relapsing back into depression or anxiety). The "dose" of exercise needed to elicit cognitive and mood benefits is small, with studies indicating that moderate intensity movement an average of three times weekly for nine weeks yields comparable antidepressant effects to medications or psychotherapy. Keep in mind that this recommendation is based on the amount shown to be effective as a "treatment" for people with depression, but even smaller amounts of movement—basically *any* amount of movement—will enhance myokine signaling across the entire gut-heart-brain axis.

Even better than simply working out in a gym is to exercise outside, especially if you can do it in a park or other natural environment. Even just taking a walk outdoors has been shown to result in significant upticks in mood, energy, focus, and overall well-being. This link between mental fitness and nature has spawned an entire subspecialty in psychology research related to the mood-boosting benefits of nature, green spaces, and, increasingly, "blue spaces" near water and coastlines. Exercising in nature seems to add an additional meditative layer to the physical movement, truly bringing the body/mind connection to bear on our mental fitness.

Being outside—whether running, walking, gardening, or doing something else—also puts us in direct contact with bacteria, which, like their relatives in our gut microbiome, can help to foster and strengthen the connections across our gut-heart-brain axis, particularly by tuning the immune system to be better at managing emotions. Some researchers believe that the steep rise in our epidemic of depression and anxiety is due largely to our growing disconnection with nature and our loss of contact with these natural bacteria.

In some cases (including many of my own personal experiences) exercising outdoors can induce a sense of wonder, awe, and consciousness-expanding that is akin to a spiritual experience. This is because of the unique cocktail of endorphins, endocannabinoids, neurotransmitters, hormones, electrical signals, and blood flow that combine in no way other than through exercise. The euphoria-inducing effects of "nature exercise" are very similar to the sensations induced by a class of natural plant-derived compounds called entheogens that have been used for centuries in traditional medicine systems (and religions) around the world. You might be familiar with some of these compounds and plants, such as hemp/marijuana (endocannabinoids), "magic" mushrooms (psilocybin), ayahuasca (dimethyltryptamine), and many others. Unique among the sensations of entheogens and the cocktail of nature-exercise compounds is one of "harmonic unity"—a sense of deep connection with nature, with other people, and with something bigger than yourself.

At this point of the book, I hope it is becoming clear that achieving your optimal state of mental fitness relies heavily on getting the *right signals* to your head brain. We can generate some of those signals directly in our head brain, but the majority of them come from other places, including our microbiome (gut brain), our electromagnetic rhythm (heart brain), our immune and inflammatory cytokines (axis), the nutrients in our food (diet), and the myokines and other exercise-induced molecules (movement). When these signals are weak or inefficient or inconsistent, we not only feel bad but our resilience is compromised and we actually lose hope. But when our signaling system is strong, robust, and reliable, we have the ability to overcome obstacles and "show up" (even to stressful situations) with energy and focus and vigor. All of that undoubtedly results in a win for each of us individually, in which we feel and perform at our best. Perhaps the very best outcome is the ripple effect, where our own enhanced mental fitness permeates out to others around us, enabling us to connect to, cooperate with, and mutually support our friends, family, coworkers, and community.

Seeing is believing. MentalFitness.tv has a series of movement videos that explain and demonstrate the seven foundational movements that we all need to keep our physical bodies working at peak function:

➤ Squat

➤ Pull

➤ Rotation

➤ Lunge

➤ Hinge

➤ Locomotion

➤ Push

CHAPTER 7

STRESS AND SLEEP

Stress and Sleep—Two Sides of a Coin

Research studies are quite clear on the fact that reducing stress helps improve sleep—just as getting better sleep helps to control stress and reduce stress hormones like cortisol. That's all well and good, but I also understand that telling you to "manage stress" is a lot easier than *actually* controlling it in your frantic life. However, you can make changes to your mindset and emotional regulation with simple (but not all easy) techniques to help you manage stress and improve resilience.

Your high levels of chronic stress put you in pretty good company. National surveys consistently show that Americans rate stress as the number one reason for a trip to the doctor, and medical surveys clearly indicate that men report to the doctor with lower back pain or fatigue (physical manifestations of stress), while women tend to report fibromyalgia or depression (mental manifestations of stress). That's not a coincidence; that's direct evidence that stressed-out lives are causing people to physically hurt and mentally feel terrible, eventually leading us away from mental fitness and toward psychological burnout.

This chapter will focus on the close links between stress and sleep, the nature of inadequate sleep as a unique stress on body and mind, and why natural approaches to improving both stress resilience and sleep quality are safer and more effective than the synthetic drugs routinely dispensed to mask depression and knock us out at night.

Often, when I give a public seminar on stress, I like to start off by holding up a glass of water and asking the audience to guess how much it weighs. People will generally call out guesses that range from eight ounces to a pound. But the point I like to make is that the actual weight of the water glass doesn't really matter. As a "stress" to my arm, the weight is less important than the duration of time that I need to hold it up. If I hold the glass for a minute or two, then it is not much of a stress at all, but if you were to ask me to hold it for an hour or a day or a week, then I'd be in trouble. It works the same way with your exposure to other stressors, such as traffic, bills, family commitments, and the millions of other little stresses you encounter day in and day out. Eventually, you will reach a breaking point unless you actively manage those stresses. Everybody—no matter how tough you think you are, no matter how resistant to stress you think you are, no matter how much you think that you thrive on stress—has a personal breaking point when it comes to stress exposure. By managing stress and getting adequate sleep as well as incorporating the other techniques, including nutrition, exercise, and dietary supple-mentation, you can continually modulate your own individual stress load and hopefully keep that "breaking point" at bay.

Okay, back to my glass of water. Let's say that I'm asked to hold the water glass for a week. Impossible, you might say. Not so. If I'm smart about managing this stress, I might be able to handle it. Maybe I can take short breaks, where I put the glass down for a few minutes each hour. Perhaps I can lessen my personal burden by asking a colleague or a friend or family member to hold the glass for a little while. Maybe I can leave the glass at work and not worry about dragging this "burden" home with me at night. Any and all of these strategies (and dozens of others) are ways in which I can manage my stress response—even if just for a few minutes. Think about some of your own sources of stress as well as some ways you can remove yourself from exposure to those stressors or off-load those stress-ors, even temporarily, to give yourself a break and a chance to recover.

A recent study by the Families and Work Institute found that one in three American workers felt chronically overworked because of technology (mostly cell phones and email that enable people to be working anywhere and everywhere, all the time). This scenario has become even more common with the COVID-19 quarantines, during which so many people started working and schooling from home, leading millions of us into the "always on and always available" status (assuming you didn't lose your job like so many millions of others, which is another level of financial stress covered later). It is really too bad that "being busy" has become such a status symbol, because it is clear from the scientific research that being too busy and always being "on" is detrimental to long-term physical health and mental fitness. Don't get me wrong—hard work is important and valuable. But working too hard for too long leads to burnout, reduced creativity, and inefficiency. It is not much of an overstatement to say that you can literally work yourself to death.

We know from studies of animals and humans that at least three factors can make a huge difference in how the body responds to a given stressor:

1. Whether the stress has any *outlet*

2. Whether the stressor is *predictable*

3. Whether the human or animal thinks it has any *control* over the stressor

These three factors—outlet, predictability, and control—emerge as modulating factors again and again in research studies of stress. For example, if you put a rat in a cage and subject it to a series of low-voltage electric shocks, the rat develops metabolic imbalances such as elevated stress hormones, blood sugar, and inflammatory markers, which lead quickly to gut problems such as ulcers and leaky gut, heart problems like hypertension, and mental problems like depression and anxiety. If you take another rat and give it the same series of shocks but also give it an outlet for its stress—such as something to chew on, something to eat, or a wheel to run on—it is able to maintain balance across biochemistry and stays physically and mentally healthy. The same is true for humans under stress. While we might refrain from chewing on anything other than a pencil (and try to avoid stress-eating that bag of chips), we can go for a run, scream at the wall, or do something else that serves as an outlet for buffering that stress.

Let's turn now to the second of the three stress modulators: predictability. Suppose someone woke you up in the middle of the night, put you on a plane, and then made you jump out of it at ten thousand feet. Pretty stressful, huh? This experience would certainly be accompanied by elevated heart rate and blood pressure, changes in blood levels of glucose and fatty acids, and, of course, a huge spike in stress hormones. What do you think would happen if you were forced to do this every other night for the next few months? Far from being a stressed-out bundle of nerves, you would actually get accustomed to it—and your stress response would become less pronounced. This scenario has actually been studied in US Army Rangers who were training at jump school to become paratroopers. At the start of training, the soldiers endured enormous increases in stress hormone levels during each jump. But by the end of the course, their stress responses were virtually nonexistent. By making the stressor more predictable (you know it is coming, and you are prepared for it), each soldier could control their stress response to a much greater degree. This "knowing it's coming" scenario is different from being worried and anxious about a potential future stressor such as losing your job, because the former is more predictable as a specific stress that you've experienced before (and can adapt to), while the latter is unknown and uncertain and thus less predictable. Uncertainty is one of the predominant drivers of human stress.

Finally, the concept of control is central to understanding why some people respond to a stressor with gigantic disruptions in metabolism while others respond to the same stressor with little more than a yawn. This idea has been demonstrated in rats that have been trained to press a lever to avoid getting shocked. Every time the rat gets shocked, it presses the lever, and the next shock is delayed for several minutes. Because the rat has some degree of control over his situation, that rat also has a lower occurrence of stress-related diseases (such as ulcers and infections). An interesting comparison can be made to people working under high-stress conditions, such as during a period of corporate layoffs. For many workers, this situation is one of high instability and low control (thus high stress), while others, perhaps those in a department that will be unaffected by job cuts or among people who have a fallback plan (such as a part-time job on the side), experience much less stress and fewer health problems.

Keep in mind that the concepts of predictability and control do not mean that you need to try to gain a high degree of control over every aspect of your life or try to see into the future to predict every possible scenario, because trying to do so can actually increase your stress and lead to anger (when you can't control everything) and anxiety (when you can't predict everything). Instead, managing stress usually means doing your best to control those things you have the power to control and accepting those things that you have little (or no) control over. We'll talk more about this concept of "going with the flow" in the next chapter.

How to "Manage" Stress

Whether you feel like you are on the verge of burnout or just a little tired from a typical twenty-first-century day, the last thing you probably want to hear is someone telling you to reduce stress. I'm right there with you; few things ratchet up my own stress levels more than someone telling me to relax (even if they are 100 percent correct). Fortunately, a multitude of research-backed and highly effective strategies for managing stress are available to you. Best of all, you do not have to drastically alter your lifestyle to implement most of them. Here are a few of my favorites that I have shared with clients and readers over the years, and I invite you to consider incorporating them into your daily routine to maintain and improve your mental fitness.

Manage your electronic interruptions.

The beeps, buzzes, or other sounds from your computer and mobile phone can add an annoying level of stress to your day. Instead of just automatically responding like a trained chimp every time you get an electronic interruption, take charge of those devices and set them to alert you only at specific times. For instance, most email programs have their default setting to check for new messages every five minutes—which means you could be interrupted by the new-message beep ninety-six times in an eight-hour day! How do you expect to get any "real" work done when you get interrupted every five minutes? This is no way to get into the creative "flow" state where you solve problems and generate breakthrough ideas or the "deep work" state where you can use your mental fitness to create meaningful value. Consider setting your email programs on your computer and phone to download emails only when you ask for them instead of pushing them to you automatically, and completely shutting off your email programs until the second half of your day, enabling you to get your important work accomplished in the morning when you're mentally fresh.

Whenever possible, leave the cell phone behind.

It may be hard to imagine today, but it wasn't too many years ago that people got along perfectly fine without cell phones. Try taking a break from your phone when possible by leaving it behind. I make that recommendation because if you carry your phone with you—even if you tell yourself that you won't answer it—a part of your mind still waits for it to chirp or buzz or play your favorite ringtone. Let that part of your brain relax and forget about the phone for a short period of time. For myself, I find that when I run with my phone (as I might do when I'm traveling and running in an unfamiliar location), my mind is not as open and creative as it is when I'm doing a "moving meditation" and running phone-free along my local trails.

Read trash.

Get a book or magazine that has no redeeming social value—and enjoy it. If this is too decadent for your tastes, then alternate a book that is "good for you" and might teach you something (like this one) with a "junk" book that you can simply lose yourself in. Why? Because it allows your mind to "escape" and recharge so it comes back even stronger, more creative, and more resilient to stress. Once, on a cross-country flight, I sat next to a woman who was reading a genetic research journal while I was reading a bicycling magazine. As a fellow scientist, I commented on her reading material, and she laughed, because underneath her research journal she had one of those celebrity gossip tabloids that you see at the grocery checkout stand. She explained that she couldn't wait to get through her genetics journal so she could catch up on the latest "dirt." It was hilarious! It turns out that we were both headed to the same research conference in Boston, and we both appreciated the importance of "getting away" for a few minutes in our "junky" books and magazines.

Take a mini-vacation every day.

One of the best ways to de-stress during your workday is to revive the lost art of lunch. Take it! Too many people skip lunch (which is bad metabolically and mentally) or gobble it down at their desks (which can be even worse). Instead, take the hour to enjoy a healthy meal and relax your mind. Even better, use that hour to visit with friends or coworkers. You'll have a more productive second half of the day and likely accomplish even more high-quality work with improved creativity and efficiency than if you had worked through lunch. And be sure to get up from your desk every hour or two for a quick stretch or walk around the office. You'll be amazed at how a quick flex of your muscles and a surge in your circulation can help clear the cobwebs from your mind.

Take a full day off each week.

No work. No thoughts about work or worries about work. Take this day to relax, reflect, and recharge (regardless of whether or not a sabbath day of rest has any religious connotations for you). Read a book. Take a walk. Luxuriate in the act of doing nothing. I guarantee that if you give yourself over to a solid month of "do-nothing Sundays" (or Saturdays, or whichever day of the week works for your schedule), you will feel more physically and mentally refreshed than you could possibly imagine. Doing nothing will give you back a lot.

Recreate to re-create.

Giving yourself permission to relax does not mean that you're a slacker; it means that you're a step ahead of the nose-to-the-grindstone automatons who are on a fast road to burnout. As a long-time nutrition consultant to some very elite-level athletes and other high-achievers, I can tell you without question that knowing when to "go hard" and when to "ease off" is what separates Olympic champions and uber-successful entrepreneurs from those who compete but fail to reach the top step of the podium. Although your own life might be "too busy" most of the time, taking those moments of relaxation and decompression is what will allow you to keep jumping back in with renewed energy and creativity.

Get a massage or take a bath.

I get it—massage can sound a little woo-woo, and hot baths don't exactly sound like they can help you accomplish more, but hear me out. Australian researchers have shown that something as simple as a fifteen-minute weekly back massage reduces stress hormone levels (cortisol) and overall measures of anxiety in a group of high-stress nurses. Another study of massage conducted at the University of Miami Miller School of Medicine showed a remarkable 31 percent reduction in cortisol levels following massage therapy as well as a 28 percent increase in the feel-good neurotransmitter serotonin (either of which would lead to a noticeable improvement in mental fitness). In similar studies, Japanese scientists in Osaka have shown a significant reduction in cortisol levels in high-stress men following the relaxing practice of traditional Japanese hot baths. The men with the highest stress levels had the most dramatic reductions in cortisol levels. These studies prove that the relaxing nature of massage and hot baths is an effective approach to maintaining biochemical balance. Even though it can sometimes feel difficult to "fit it in" in terms of time management and the feeling that I really should be doing some "real" work, the one-hour massage that I get every other week and the thirty-minute hot tub soak that I get a few times per week (especially after skiing) pay back compounded dividends in terms of physical health and mental fitness.

Imagine creative solutions.

Japanese researchers in Kyoto have shown that guided-imagery exercises (relaxing by imagining solutions to stress) can help people reduce cortisol, glucose, and anxiety levels after the very first session. In a series of studies, subjects practiced replacing unpleasant mental images of stressful events (such as you having an argument with your boss) with comfortable thoughts (such as you having a thoughtful and engaging discussion with your boss), resulting in a displacement of stress and a shift toward a balanced emotional state. Psychology researchers at UCLA have also shown that stressed patients who performed a "value-affirmation task"—where you mentally recite your personal values and itemize the things that are most important to you—were able to short-circuit stress and anxiety responses in reaction to stressful events.

Get away for a long weekend.

Even short periods of "getting away" can result in significant drops in cortisol, stress, and anxiety, with corresponding elevations in serotonin, oxytocin, dopamine, and overall vigor (mental fitness). In one study, a three-day, two-night weekend getaway trip resulted in a decrease in cortisol levels and overall inflammatory stress markers as well as a boost in immune system function—suggesting that a mini-vacation is good for our mental fitness as well as our physical health. It doesn't have to be expensive or exotic; it just has to be "away" enough to get you out of your hectic daily routine—to see something new and unexpected.

Take a yoga class.

Swedish psychologists have shown that ten sessions of yoga over four weeks resulted in significant psychological (mental fitness) and physiological (physical fitness) benefits in men and women. Participants in the yoga sessions showed improvements in their levels of cortisol, stress, anger, exhaustion, and blood pressure.

Pray.

Regardless of how you feel about religion or spirituality, research shows that prayer can have a highly significant positive impact on both physical health and mental fitness. One study on religion by researchers at Arizona State University has shown that people who are more spiritual and pray more often have lower cortisol levels, lower blood pressure, lower anxiety, and higher stress resilience. Part of this effect appears to be related to the stress factors described earlier (outlet/predictability/control), whereby prayer helps us understand that not everything is within our control and some things are "in God's hands" and need to be accepted and dealt with (more on this idea of "control" in the next chapter).

Get a pet.

For some people, stress management may come on four legs. Scientists at Virginia Commonwealth University found that high-stress health-care professionals were able to significantly lower their stress and anxiety levels after as little as five minutes of "dog therapy." Follow-up research has confirmed the same benefits for physical and mental health, leading to therapy dogs becoming a fairly mainstream intervention to help people deal with the stress of cancer treatment, postsurgical recovery, and a wide range of psychological treatments, including recovery from drug addictions. As a dog owner myself, I can attest to the curative powers of my fur-babies as a buffer against stress and a pathway toward calm (I'd also like to think that they get similar benefits from the belly rubs, but they are no good at completing my psychological surveys).

Tune in to tunes.

According to a number of studies, listening to relaxing music can reduce cortisol and stress levels significantly faster following a stressful event compared to sitting in silence. Numerous studies have shown that upbeat music can significantly improve exercise performance (extending both endurance and strength in different studies by as much as 20 percent) and reduce pain perception (as effectively as over-the-counter and prescription pain drugs). Listening to background music (such as the soundtrack at your local coffee shop) has also been shown to improve creativity and work performance (again, compared to working in silence)—so there are ample physical and mental benefits to cranking up the tunes.

Believe in yourself.

Remember the story of *The Little Engine That Could*? Well, young children show marked resilience to stress when they apply the same "I think I can" approach to school stressors as the little train did in its attempt to climb the hill in the classic tale. In a study by Swedish researchers, school kids had reduced stress responses when they approached stressful situations with mental imagery that affirmed "I can solve this task." The same is true for adults, but to be most effective, we need to be a little more nuanced and deliberate than just "thinking happy thoughts." We can use positive affirmations as a strategic mental fitness tool.

One of the most effective ways to weave positive affirmations into your daily routine is to have a "trigger" for when you practice each one—such as when you wake up, when you take your first sip of coffee, when you are brushing your teeth, when you are in the shower, when you sit down to eat something, when you go to the bathroom, whenever you are standing in line or waiting on hold or stopped at a traffic light, and when you go to bed at night. Here are a few examples:

■ WAKE UP

Use a positive affirmation to set the tone for the day, such as "I am calm and peaceful today" or "I exude balance and patience." Focusing on your intention for the day and accompanied by a few deep breaths, you are using your conscious mind to establish an unconscious pattern for the rest of the day—a pattern that you will reinforce with the steps that follow.

▪ COFFEE

Don't just gulp down your morning coffee (or tea or whatever your beverage of choice might be) as a jolt of caffeine, but rather intentionally bring your focus to the attributes of the beverage. Consider the aroma of the coffee brewing, the warmth of your cup, the bitterness or sweetness or creaminess in your mouth (depending on how you take your coffee). These simple thoughts take mere seconds, but they allow us to focus on the simple pleasures of life and away from the buzzing in our heads. You can also take this moment to express gratitude, which we will also revisit in more detail as a nightly bedtime routine.

▪ BRUSH TEETH

When you're brushing your teeth in the morning, think about "cleaning" your thoughts as you clean your teeth. This technique of going into the day with a clean slate, no matter what happened yesterday, and not prejudging any situation as good or bad can remind us to be open to new possibilities and experiences—to be nonresistant and receptive to whatever the day may bring. This openness fosters our ability to learn, to see connections, and to solve problems that may be closed off to us when we are locked in a mindset dominated by stress.

▪ SHOWER

We can take the "clean teeth/clean slate" a step further, to actively wash away specific negative thoughts and reactions. For example, while you are in the shower, think of a negative thought as a dirt residue—as dust clinging to your skin—and then imagine the warm water and suds washing it off and down the drain. This technique is particularly effective for things that are out of our control, such as the reactions that other people have to events. We can control only our own actions and reactions, not the actions and reactions of other people, so we need to not worry about those and let them wash away.

■ EAT

The concept of "diet" as used in this book refers to much more than just the food we eat and the nutrients we consume. It refers to our "habitual exposure" and our consumption of food, of thoughts, of energy, and of all forms of "information" coming into our gut, brain, and heart. This is why I like to use the occasion of a meal to integrate the actual nutrients of the food with physical and mental inputs—as an opportunity for us to internalize positive energy. Before and after you eat your food (which is hopefully more often a healthy salad than it is a fast-food hamburger), try a quick physical and mental prep where you actually shake your arms and legs (physical prep) and deep breathe in and out a few times (mental prep). If you've ever watched the start of the Olympic 100-meter dash, you have seen that before the sprinters enter their starting blocks, they shake out their arms and legs and then crouch into the blocks and take a few cleansing breaths before settling into their start position. At this point, they are in a place of physical and mental calm, and they are ready to perform. We don't want to think of what comes next—eating and enjoying our meal—as something that we want to sprint through (we actually want to eat mindfully), but the principle of preparing sets off an anti-stress ripple effect that improves our digestion and assimilation of nutrients as well as our mental fitness in the moment.

■ BATHROOM

For a lot of us, bathroom breaks throughout the day are some of the few times we truly have to ourselves—don't waste them by checking Twitter! This is a perfect time to use these precious few minutes for breath work, which is nearly universally regarded by monks, gurus, shamans, scientists, and physicians as both calming and invigorating. This does not have to be complicated or structured like a formal 5-5-5 type of mindful meditation breathwork; it can be as simple as taking a few deep inhalations and exhalations.

■ WAITING

It is so easy to get extremely irritated by even the slightest little delay or inconvenience—even when we're asked to wait for mere seconds. However, we can easily replace the irritation of waiting on hold or standing in line or sitting at a red light with positive thoughts and affirmations for the well-being of others (which simultaneously improves our own well-being). The next chapter outlines a specific type of meditation known as loving-kindness meditation that we can use whenever we're waiting—instead of whipping out our phones to check the news or send a text—where you basically send out "good vibes" to other people. This simple practice of wishing for the grocery cashier to have a stress-free day, that the driver of the car in front of you has a safe commute, and the customer service rep receives more thanks than complaints for solving her callers' inquiries helps us mentally connect to other people and induces a neurological and biochemical calming effect in ourselves.

■ OUTSIDE

Whenever you go outside—even if it's just to walk from your house to your car for the daily commute or from your car into the office for the workday—it's important to look up at the sky and consider for just a moment how incredibly lucky you are to be part of this amazing, infinite, connected universe. The emotion of "awe" (which I cover in more detail in the next chapter) is one of the most effective emotional states for reducing anxiety and depression while boosting resilience and mental fitness. The more often we can induce our sense of vastness and expansiveness and interconnectedness—even if just for a few moments each day—the more we are able to put our own personal struggles and stresses in context.

■ BED

One of the most studied and most effective ways to calm anxious thoughts, alleviate depression, and stimulate mental fitness is to express gratitude. While expressing gratitude can be effective any time, it seems to be particularly effective as a regular nighttime routine before turning in for bed. The trick with a regular nightly gratitude practice is to "think small," because expressing gratitude for the little things is a proven way to focus our minds away from negative thoughts and ruminations on problems toward positive emotions and joy. Little things might include your gratitude that you have a bed to sleep in and a roof over your head; it might be the snoring dog on the floor; it might be that funny text you got from a friend, or the cat video that you saw online; or it might even be that this horrible day is over and you have a "redo" coming in eight hours. Cultivating an "attitude of gratitude" might sound hokey—especially when you have a lot of crap to deal with every day—but in all the research into psychological well-being, this is the technique that rises to the top again and again as being the most effective and simplest to implement to help reduce anxiety, stress, and depression while also improving myriad aspects of physical health and mental fitness, including sleep quality.

Poor Sleep as a Unique Form of Stress

Easily the most effective stress-management technique you can practice is really very simple: get enough sleep! Even one or two nights of good, sound, restful sleep can do more for maintaining your biochemical balance (stress hormones, blood sugar, inflammation) and improving your mental fitness than just about any other intervention. It is almost impossible to overstate the crucial role that adequate sleep plays in controlling your stress response, helping you lose weight, boosting your energy levels, improving your mood, and, of course, bolstering your resilience and elevating your mental fitness.

Because sleep is such an important component for building mental fitness, I'm devoting the rest of the chapter to it. I've written in previous chapters about the "stress" of poor diet and sedentary lifestyle on the function and structure of our entire gut-heart-brain axis. This chapter considers how the things we typically think of as "stress" do the same. These various types of stressors can all impact our mental fitness in various ways. On a certain level, most of us will be aware that eating a doughnut is not as healthy for us as eating an apple—and that the doughnut is creating a certain level of stress on our system. The same applies for sitting on the couch versus going for a walk and for being tense and irritated versus being calm and relaxed in any given situation. However, most of us don't have an appreciation for the extremely high level of stress that inadequate sleep delivers to body and mind. Many of us think that we can get by with inadequate sleep, at least for a while, but that thinking is completely wrong. Lack of sleep is perhaps the most underappreciated—and most toxic—sources of stress in our modern lives. Sleep is one of the most important and most modifiable of all the lifestyle factors associated with mental fitness. We need to "consume" enough sleep every night to rejuvenate our brains, to allow our bodies to recover and repair, to consolidate memories, and to test out emotional scenarios (more on all of these to follow). If we "starve" ourselves of proper sleep—either in quantity or quality—we suffer in myriad ways, from minor things such as fatigue and short temper to major things such as increased risk for cancer, diabetes, and Alzheimer's disease.

There are many reasons why we don't get enough sleep—and why we fail to appreciate the health implications. One is that our modern overstimulated world often seems perfectly designed to prevent good sleep. Another is that most of us are simply unaware of our sleep patterns (we're unconscious, after all). Just as you pay little attention to the fact that your heart beats in a regular pattern, so too are you normally unaware of your body's natural rhythm during restful sleep. But night after night, your body follows a well-worn path into dreamland: Breathing slows, muscles relax, heart rate and blood pressure drop, and body temperature falls. The brain releases the "sleep hormone," melatonin, and begins a slow descent into sleep. The rapid beta waves of your restless wakeful state in the daytime gradually change into the slower alpha waves that are characteristic of calm wakefulness, or "relaxed alertness," where you generally want to spend most of your time. Eventually, your brain drops into the still-slower theta waves that predominate during the various stages of sleep.

During a full night of sleep, we normally pass through several stages: Stage 0 is when we are awake. Stages 1 and 2 are "light sleep" (lasting ten to fifteen minutes). Stage 3 is "deep sleep" (lasting another five to fifteen minutes). Finally, we enter the deepest portion of sleep in stage 4 (lasting about thirty minutes). Even though stage 4 lasts only about a half hour, it is the most "famous" portion of the sleep cycle, because it is when you dream and exhibit rapid eye movement, popularly referred to as REM. Your total sleep cycle, from early stages 1 and 2 to final REM sleep, takes an average of ninety minutes to complete. And, most importantly for people who have trouble sleeping, this cycle repeats itself over and over throughout the night, which means that interruptions can make it harder to get back to sleep, depending on which part of the cycle you're in when awakened.

Bright Days and Dark Nights

Perhaps the most dominant driver of our twenty-four-hour day/night circadian rhythm is exposure to light in the day and darkness at night. But our modern world easily and frequently interrupts our natural wake/sleep patterns with bright lights, television screens, and smartphones. On the flip side, we can actually use different levels of light exposure during the day and night to "set us up" for a good night of sleep. For example, we can try getting out in the bright sunlight to encourage daytime serotonin production and try sleeping in a very dark bedroom to encourage nighttime melatonin production. Having some daytime exposure to bright light can not only improve sleep that night, but it also improves mood during that day and can even enhance immune function and speed wound healing (both benefits due to a lot more than just the superior vitamin D levels associated with sunlight exposure). Today, most of us spend too much time in twilight—not bright enough in the day and too bright in the evening. Light "strength" (referred to as *illuminance*) is measured in lux units and refers to the amount of light striking a surface. Studies of agricultural and other "off-grid" societies, such as the Amish, have shown that lux exposure can range from around 4,000 in the summer daytime (compared to about 600 for the average office worker) while winter daytime values drop to around 1,500 for the Amish (and way down to about 200 for the modern office worker). During the evening, the average illuminance in Amish homes is only about 10 lux, while the average modern electrified home is at least five to ten times higher, around 50–100 lux.

It isn't just that bright light is bad or that darkness is good for sleep. The *amplitude between* the two extremes is crucial to establish and maintain healthy circadian rhythms. We need to experience a marked contrast in lux exposure (which can range from 10,000 lux of daylight to 1 lux of deep twilight to 0.001 lux of dark night). These fluctuations in light/dark exposure are sensed by our eyes, transmitted to our head brain, and influence our body clock, sleep patterns, mood, alertness, and every aspect of our mental fitness and physical health. Our eyes contain light-responsive cells called retinal ganglion cells (RGCs) that are particularly sensitive to light in the blue part of the spectrum, which includes bright daylight but also light from screens, such as televisions, computers, and smartphones. Our RGCs send blue light signals to the part of the brain that controls alertness (our body's master clock, the suprachiasmatic nucleus, or SCN) so that even just an hour of exposure to low-intensity blue light increases alertness as much as drinking two cups of coffee. This is why looking at your smartphone before bed often interferes with restful sleep—because the blue light signals your brain that it is day rather than night. Studies have shown that people living in areas with high levels of light pollution (such as cities) tend to go to bed later than those living in darker areas (such as rural areas) and also have fewer total hours of sleep, have higher reports of daytime fatigue, and have lower scores for sleep quality and overall quality of life.

Understanding how light and dark exposure influences our daytime moods and nighttime sleep can help us to establish a regimen to harness these signals to improve our mental fitness. For example, studies have shown that if you can expose yourself to daytime light, such as by sitting next to a window at work or taking a walk outside at lunch, you're likely to sleep better at night (falling asleep faster, waking up less often, and sleeping deeper) and also feel better the following day (with higher indices for mood, alertness, energy, and reaction times). These findings are starting to be used in hospitals (to enhance healing and recovery) and nursing homes (to improve mood and cognitive function).

Sleep Loss Damages Our Three Brains

If you're not yet convinced of the mental fitness benefits of adequate sleep, consider that few people fully appreciate that lack of sleep is one of the most important determinants of whether you might get Alzheimer's disease in the future! Even a single night of poor sleep can lead to brain changes similar to the damage seen in Alzheimer's patients, with a buildup of the beta-amyloid protein plaques that are normally flushed out by the brain's glymphatic "housekeeping" system after a good night of sleep.

Our gut microbiome also seems to exhibit certain circadian patterns that may be related to light/dark cycles and to food timing—such as when we eat breakfast, how long we fast overnight, whether or not we have a midnight snack—which suggests that we can target the gut brain to encourage our head brain to get a good night of sleep. A recent study from researchers in Florida showed that overall microbiome diversity was correlated with overall sleep quality in a bidirectional fashion, suggesting that a resilient and diverse microbiome helps us sleep and that high-quality sleep helps us maintain a healthy microbiome and proper signaling across the entire gut-brain axis (including our immune system and inflammatory network). For example, better sleep was associated with improved levels of microbiome bacteria species in the Bacteroidetes phyla, which produce gamma-aminobutyric acid (GABA) and serotonin (neurotransmitters that promote mood, relaxation, and sleep). Higher levels of Bacteroidetes have also been associated with improved metabolism and weight loss, suggesting that one of the ways that good sleep promotes weight loss (which has been shown in dozens of recent studies) is via the microbiome.

Because sleep problems are at epidemic levels, millions of people look to a pharmaceutical solution: using sleep drugs to knock them out at night. But not only is this not particularly effective in the short-term, it is potentially extremely dangerous in the long-term. Sleep drugs—Ambien in particular and benzodiazepines like Valium in general—have been linked to longer duration of sleep (they knock you out for more hours compared to a placebo) but not to improved sleep quality. In fact, these drugs will actually enhance your brain's ability to consolidate *negative* emotional memories during sleep, so you're likely to wake up with a higher level of agitation, tension, and stress—or precisely the opposite outcome you were hoping for. And because sleep drugs fail to produce natural sleep patterns, their prolonged use is also associated with higher risk for a long list of diseases, including Alzheimer's, diabetes, and certain cancers.

The Food and Drug Administration requires sleep drugs to carry the agency's most stringent and prominent safety warning (the "black box" warning) to call attention to possible side effects, including serious injuries or death. Even the lowest doses of all of the major sleep drugs are required to carry this warning, including Ambien (zolpidem), Lunesta (eszopiclone), and Sonata (zaleplon).

How Much Sleep Do You Need?

In sleep-research labs—where alarm clocks, lights, and other interruptions can be banished—scientists have found that the natural duration allowing adequate "cycling" through the sleep stages described earlier (the "physiological ideal") is eight hours and fifteen minutes. We've known this for decades, and research studies have confirmed the "eight-hour rule" on numerous occasions. Yet according to the Centers for Disease Control and Prevention, more than half of Americans still get less than seven hours of sleep on a regular basis.

The idea of getting more than eight hours of sleep per night may sound great—but what if you simply can't (or won't) get that much shut-eye? You could be setting yourself up for numerous health problems, beginning with the fact that your blood sugar levels will rise. Sleep researchers have shown that getting only four to six hours of sleep per night results in signs of impaired glucose tolerance and insulin resistance. This means that cheating on sleep—even for only a few nights—can put a person in a prediabetic state. These changes in insulin action and blood sugar control are also linked to an increase in risk for inflammation-related conditions, such as heart disease. Poor sleep also contributes to obesity, because it precipitates changes on the hormonal level. Growth hormone and leptin are reduced in people who spend less time in deep sleep. Leptin is a hormone that plays important roles in regulating appetite, body weight, and metabolism. When you have less growth hormone in your system, it typically results in a loss of muscle and a gain of fat over time. Reduced levels of leptin will lead to hunger and carbohydrate cravings.

In a famous (and cruel) series of animal studies in the 1980s, researchers showed that rats subjected to total sleep deprivation started to die by day eleven without sleep. By thirty-two days, all of the animals deprived of sleep were deceased even though there was no clear biological cause of death. The animals simply "gave out," probably through a combination of physical and mental breakdowns involving the brain and the immune system. Fast forward four decades, and we know that sleep is when our brain "cleans" itself by flushing out accumulated toxins of the day. It's when our body secretes anabolic hormones to stimulate tissue and organ repairs. It's when our immune system hits the reset button and learns how to fine-tune its vigilance for the next day of exposures.

Given all these health impacts, I am continually astonished by how many people think they can just "get by" with inadequate sleep and are then surprised when they struggle with low energy, belly fat, constant cravings, brain fog, low sex drive, depression, or any of the other problems associated with being underslept, overstressed, and out of biochemical balance. Thinking that you can "get by" with inadequate sleep is exactly like thinking you can "get by" with a steady diet of Twinkies.

Sadly, trying to "make up" for missed sleep is also not an effective option, with recent studies showing that the metabolic damage of sleep loss can't be reversed by extra sleep later on. For example, researchers at the University of Colorado showed that sleeping five hours nightly during the week led to the expected derangements in insulin sensitivity, blood sugar balance, evening snacking, and belly fat gain. But they also found that sleeping in on the weekend (as many hours as they wanted) not only didn't help restore normal metabolism, but the sleep-deprived subjects also had even worse metabolism numbers and snacking behaviors compared to the "normal sleep" group getting eight to nine hours nightly. If you're shorting yourself on sleep, you are virtually guaranteeing that your biochemical balance will be chronically disrupted, and you are putting yourself in a position of weak mental fitness.

To give you some idea of just how detrimental a lack of sleep can be to your biochemical balance and mental fitness, consider what happens to an average fifty-year-old who sleeps just six hours per night. That middle-aged person has evening cortisol levels more than twelve times higher than the average thirty-year-old who sleeps eight hours per night!

Not only will an inadequate quality or quantity of sleep upset stress hormone balance but it will also limit your ability to fall asleep the next night (because your cortisol is still too high) as well as the amount of time that your mind spends in the most restful stages of deep sleep. A vicious cycle gets set into motion when you experience poor sleep: an overactive stress response and subtle changes in signaling across the gut-heart-brain axis that lead you down the path away from mental fitness and toward burnout.

Even though numerous research studies verify the damage caused by sleep deprivation, and even if you now understand the importance of sleep for our mental fitness and performance across our gut-heart-brain axis, you may feel lucky to get just six or seven hours of nightly shut-eye. I know I do, and yet I also realize this is still not enough sleep to maintain my own mental fitness. On top of that, I also know that some of the best ways to ensure a restful night of sleep are to avoid caffeine after noon (yet I sit here writing this with an afternoon cup of java next to the laptop), leave work at the office (yet I'm writing this from my home office), and skip the late-night TV (yet all the on-demand streaming services allow me to easily binge on the latest shows), so that's three strikes for me. I tell you these personal details in the hope that you will see that maintaining and improving our mental fitness is not an all-or-nothing proposition. No one does this perfectly, myself included! Sometimes you have lots of stress, and sometimes you have less. Sometimes you get adequate sleep, but for many of us, that doesn't happen often enough. On certain days you'll be able to exercise and eat right and relax, and on other days you'll hit the drive-through and feel like you're working frantically. The point here is not to strive to be "perfect" in your efforts toward better mental fitness; rather, the best approach is to apply the principles outlined in this book as consistently as possible to ensure that you can do as much as possible to keep your mental fitness high as often as possible.

As such, please think of the suggestions below for building better sleep habits as a "buffet" rather than as a to-do list—where you can choose the things that look best to you, but don't feel like you need to try them all. Many of these tips have worked for me personally, so I try to incorporate them as often as possible.

Build a Better Bedtime

Exercise on a regular basis.

Exercise can help reduce inflammation, stress hormones, blood sugar, and simply help us feel better because of the pleasant postexercise fatigue that can help us sink into our bed in the evening.

Don't exercise too close to bedtime.

While exercise is great for the reasons just described, exercising too close to bedtime can increase alertness enough in some people to interfere with their ability to fall asleep.

Relax before bed.

Take time to unwind by enjoying a nonelectronic relaxing activity, such as reading. Electronics, including computers, video games, and televisions, can increase alertness and stimulate the brain into a wakeful state that can make it hard to fall asleep.

Make your bedroom dark and cool and (somewhat) quiet.

The slow drop in body temperature that you experience in a cool room can help you feel sleepy, and a darkened room with as little light distraction as possible can help you stay asleep. The idea of making your "room a tomb"—as dark and cool as possible (between sixty and sixty-seven degrees)—can be enhanced with a fan that provides both cooling and white noise. White noise is simply a consistent noise that comes out evenly across all the hearable frequencies, from low to high. When a noise wakes you up at night, it's not the noise itself but rather the sudden change or inconsistencies that your brain notices to jolt you awake. White noise masks these changes to help you fall asleep easier, and you wake up less frequently in the night because it keeps you from hearing *changes* in sound. I use a fan at home and a white noise app on my phone (ocean waves and rainstorms) when traveling.

If you can't fall asleep after twenty minutes, get up.

If you try to fall asleep and can't, get up and do something relaxing, such as reading, until you feel tired enough to fall asleep. The stress that comes from trying to "force" yourself to fall asleep will almost certainly keep you awake longer and may interfere with restful sleep when you finally do drift off.

Brighten your day and darken your night.

Building on our discussion earlier about the importance of bright sunlight exposure during the day and dark exposure during the night, it makes sense for all of us to apply this new science to our own pattern of brighter days and darker nights to enhance our mental fitness. Your daytime setup should include some exercise (at least four to six hours before bed), ideally done outside in bright sunlight. Your nighttime setup is to cut the caffeine after noon (because caffeine's stimulating effects can linger for five to six hours in most people) and banish blue light from television, computer, and smartphone screens at least one hour before lights out.

Find your personal wind-down routine.

It's difficult to overemphasize the importance of establishing a nightly "wind-down" routine. Each of the "build a better bedtime" techniques are effective on their own, but linking them together in a pattern that you engage in on a regular/typical basis will also help signal your brain that "we're getting ready to sleep." You'll find that falling asleep, staying asleep, and getting high-quality sleep will eventually become more of the rule than the exception.

Here is my own personal wind-down routine that I practice almost every night. Feel free to use it as a guide:

➤ **9:00 p.m.** I relax and have a snack.

- We typically watch the early local news and then stream an episode of one of the late-night comedians like Seth Meyers, John Oliver, or Trevor Noah. Your brain needs thirty to sixty minutes to wind down before bed, so being able to "disconnect" like this is a lot more effective than closing out those last few emails and then trying to immediately go to sleep.

- To keep you asleep, you need good blood sugar control, so having a small protein/carb snack like nuts/fruit, cheese/crackers, yogurt/granola can facilitate that process (but a large meal or high-calorie snack like an ice cream sundae can interfere with your sleep).

- On most nights of the week, I have a glass of wine with dinner, and on some nights I might have another glass while relaxing. My limit is two because more than that is likely to interfere with proper sleep cycling and interrupt the most restful deep stages of sleep. Sometimes, instead of a glass of wine, I'll have a cup of herbal tea. Chamomile helps relax the smooth muscle in the gut, which sends a similar relaxation signal to the brain to help us wind down.

➤ **10:00 p.m.** This is my target for going upstairs to bed.

- While I'm brushing my teeth, I think of a few things for which I am grateful. This two- to three-minute "gratitude practice" is triggered by my nightly oral hygiene routine, so I never miss it (more on mindfulness practices and triggers in the next chapter).

- After I brush my teeth, I take my evening supplements (detailed in chapter 9), which religiously includes corn grass extract to help improve sleep quality (by up to 40 percent) and omega-3s (to help balance inflammation and enhance overnight tissue repair).

- Read! This is my secret weapon for a good night of high-quality sleep. If I have completed an effective "daytime setup" (exercise in the sunlight, relax before bed, small snack), then I'll often start to get the "head bobs" after ten to fifteen minutes of reading my book (either a paper book or a Kindle to minimize blue light exposure) in my dim room (just a bedside light bright enough to read by) with a fan blowing cool air and soft white noise toward my bed.

- If, for whatever reason, my mind is still at work and I'm having trouble shutting it off, I'll do a set of deep breaths and a quick body scan—progressively relaxing each part of my body from toes to feet to calves, all the way up to my head. This simple process activates the PNS and engages our natural relaxation response. If you often have trouble shutting off the noise in your head, then keep a notebook by your bed so you can download any invasive thoughts out of your head and onto the page. This can help you stop worrying and ruminating because those thoughts will be there in the morning for you to pick back up if needed.

- If I can't fall asleep in twenty to thirty minutes, I don't stress out. I'll simply get up, grab a glass of water, write down anything that might be on my mind and interfering with my ability to relax, and then do something else (like read) until I'm more tired.

➤ **6:00 to 7:00 a.m.** This would be my target range for waking up to ensure a solid eight hours of high-quality sleep. When I'm doing it right, I'll typically wake up before my alarm clock—or before the dogs bark for their breakfast.

This is the wind-down routine that I have found works very well for me. While it, or at least certain aspects of it, might also work for you, it is important for you to find the right combination of steps and strategies that represents the best fit for your own likes and dislikes. Without exaggeration, I can tell you that having a consistent pattern of high-quality sleep can literally change your life by improving your mental fitness and physical performance across every parameter that you can imagine. Sleep is every bit as important for overall health and well-being as proper diet and regular physical activity—and just a few of these simple steps, applied consistently night after night for a few days to a few weeks, will deliver benefits for years to come.

CHAPTER 8

MINDSET

It is appropriate that I am writing this chapter on mindset during the COVID-19 pandemic and the quarantines of 2020. If there was ever a time when we all need mental fitness, it is now.

Rather than embracing the common phrase "social distancing," I've been encouraging people to practice physical distancing to slow the spread of the virus. This minor but important nuance helps people understand that we need to stay physically apart for physical health (to slow infection rates), but we also need to maintain our close social connections to maintain our mental fitness. We can still remain socially connected while being physically apart by using our phones, video chat, and various social media platforms to encourage and support one another through these chaotic and uncertain times.

Up to this point in the book, we have explored the idea that how we feel is not just in our head; it's also in our gut and microbiome and heart and immune system. It is the coordinated actions across the entire gut-heart-brain axis that ultimately determines how we feel and perform.

But that is not to say that our thoughts don't matter, because they actually matter a great deal. Remember that our use of the word *diet* in the Mental Fitness Diet refers as much to the thoughts that we feed to our head as to the food that we feed to our gut and the exercise that we feed to our heart.

When we talk about mindset, we are simply referring in a general way to the established set of attitudes someone holds. There are a zillion ways to think about how we think, but I want to focus our discussion on one particularly well-researched aspect of mindset that relates directly to mental fitness, referred to as an abundant or growth mindset. Someone with an abundant/growth mindset is an optimist who is genuinely happy for others when they achieve success, and they have a perspective that they can also improve themselves and their skills beyond wherever they are currently. Conversely, those with a scarcity or fixed mindset tend to be hypercompetitive and resent the success of other people while also feeling as if their skills are fixed as being good at certain things and bad at others. Your mindset type can not only significantly affect your ability to see the glass as half full or half empty (optimism versus pessimism) but also your perception of whether or not you can be effective in filling or draining the glass even more (growth versus fixed) or sharing some of the water with others or keeping it to yourself (abundance versus scarcity).

Your Story

Our mindset—our established set of attitudes—starts with the story we tell ourselves about who we are, where we came from, and where we are going. Your story might be positive or negative, it might be clear or muddled, it might be true or embellished, but whatever form your story takes, it is yours. We all have—and *need*—one. Making your story as clear as possible is a good place to start, because all our stories are "in progress." We are literally adding lines and chapters to them every minute of every day, and we need to know where we are if we want to plan the next step toward where we are going.

Let me give you a personal example of my own story. I was born in 1967 to an unwed mother who refused to hand her newborn son over to the nuns at the Catholic hospital. I never knew my biological father, and the man who eventually married my mother and became the dad that I grew up with was an uneducated and violent drug user and dealer. He was a high school dropout who frequently beat my mother and got my younger brother to start using drugs, ultimately resulting in my brother's overdose death in 2001. Not a great start, but I was very lucky that my mother was extremely intelligent ("wicked smaht," as we would say growing up near Boston). Even though she herself had only a couple years of college (having dropped out when she got pregnant with me), she always encouraged me to do well in school and to read and be curious about everything. I was also very lucky that some of my teachers noticed my curiosity and bumped me into the "advanced" classes, where I fell in with a group of kids who are still my closest friends to this day.

This put me on the path where I was expected to go to college, even if I didn't know how to pay for tuition on the salaries of an auto mechanic (Dad) and school bus driver (Mom). Thank goodness for scholarships and student loans, because college and graduate school were transformative for me—from studying sports medicine (BS) and fitness management (BA) at Marietta College, exercise science (MS) at the University of Massachusetts, nutritional biochemistry (PhD) at Rutgers, and entrepreneurship (EMP) at MIT to competing in rowing (collegiate and US Nationals, Olympic Festival, US National Team), cycling (collegiate and Olympic Training Center), and triathlon (professional and Team USA). My academic education and competitive sports experience have instilled in me the importance of combining knowing and understanding (the thinking part) with actively trying (the doing part)—and when something doesn't quite work out, figuring out why and trying again with a different approach. Without the influences of certain high school teachers and college coaches, I shudder to think about where I might have ended up (I'm looking at you, Barbara Leary at Amesbury High School, and you, Tom Stephanik at Marietta College).

All of that leads me up to where I am today as a deliriously happily married father of two very intelligent and grounded young adults. I was lucky to meet my wife right in the middle of my studies. We've been together now for longer than we've been apart—true soul mates—and like Forrest Gump said, we go together "like peas and carrots."

All of this is to say that I am a firm believer, as well as a prime example, that coming from meager beginnings is of less importance than moving forward with the right mindset of optimism, abundance, and growth. As a successful author (this is my fourteenth book) and product developer (having formulated hundreds of successful nutrition products), I don't have any illusions of having accomplished any of what I have by myself with just the power of positive thinking—far from it. But my mindset has enabled me to be open to lucky circumstances, to be inclined to take risks by trying something new that might not work, and to be accepting of failure as merely having learned one way not to do something before figuring out another way to try again.

What is *your* story? You probably have at least a vague idea of the formative events in your own personal narrative, but I would really encourage you to take a few minutes (or a whole afternoon) to sit down and write out your story as I have done above. Think about your story from different perspectives—certainly from your own perspective but also from the perspective of what other people might say about you. For example, I've written my story above from my own perspective and through my own lens (which is logical), but if you were to ask some of the people who read my books or use my nutrition products about me, they might say, "He's a brilliant scientist." If you were to ask some of my teammates about me, they might say, "He's a gritty competitor." If you were to ask my wife or kids about me, they might say, "He's a total goofball." Each of these other perspectives is true—but only partially so. You get the idea: the same set of circumstances viewed through different lenses or perspectives can lead to slightly different interpretations, but *you* get to decide which version makes it into your story.

There are lots of other ways to help us construct our story. One is to consider writing your own obituary. What would people say about you when you are gone, and what would you want them to say? Another is to consider what optimist and business consultant Simon Sinek calls your "why." It's a focus on why you do what you do and not simply on what you do. Yet another approach is to think about how you would describe what you want to be known for in a single sentence. Mine would be something along the lines of "he helped millions of people improve their mental fitness and enhance the lives of those around them." Granted, a single sentence needs to leave a lot of stuff out, but that is the point. The entire exercise of writing your why or your sentence or your story (or all of them) is to focus, clarify, and refine your thinking so you can think about the most important part. what comes next. That can help us determine the most beneficial thoughts and beliefs to feed our brain.

Take Action

I like to think of mindset (attitudes, or what we think) as the first part of our "what comes next" equation. The second part of the equation is the action—basically what are we going to *do* with these attitudes—or what I refer to as your *actset*. Too many people mistakenly think that they need to wait to take action until they are ready or motivated or until they feel like it. In fact, the opposite is often true: *attitude follows action!* If you can get moving, even if it is initially in the wrong direction and you need to pivot slightly, your attitude is strengthened.

Just as bad is the situation where many people are mentally ready and motivated to take action, but they are waiting for permission to get started. Permission from who? Give yourself permission to write that book (without waiting for a publisher) or start that business (without waiting for an investor) or do anything that you've been thinking about trying. After all, none of us will ever know what we are capable of until we try. So start!

Being mentally fit means having the right mindset (thinking) but also an orientation and predisposition toward action (doing). This is not to say that you should blindly run off into oblivion—you don't need to jump out of the airplane and build your parachute on the way down—but you do need to do something. One way to nudge yourself in the right direction is to take the improv approach, which encourages us to think like actors in an improvisational theater. In improv, the default position is "Yes, and." It means that we accept whatever situation is thrown at us ("yes") rather than rejecting it ("no"), and then we build on that situation to improve it to another level ("and") rather than trying to offer an alternative ("but"). You can apply this "Yes, and" technique to any situation in your life, whether personal, business, or family. This is important, because we often don't get to choose the initial situation, and we often have little to no control over certain circumstances. We just have to say yes rather than futilely rage against the injustice of the universe. What we *can* control is what comes next (the "and")—our response and actions that will help us move beyond this situation.

What Is in Our Control?

> *Be scared. You can't help that. But don't be afraid.*
> —William Faulkner

❧

> *You have power over your mind—not outside events.*
> *Realize this, and you will find strength.*
> —Marcus Aurelius

For many years, I have adopted a daily practice of Stoic philosophy that has helped me deal with trials and tribulations both large and small. It is overly simplistic to try to define Stoicism in a single sentence, but I'll try to do that anyway: it is an ancient Greek philosophy designed to help us be more resilient, happier, and more mentally fit through control over our emotions and our reactions to external events. There is a great deal of nuance with the interpretation and practice of Stoicism, so I invite you to learn more at DailyStoic.com, in the books by Ryan Holiday, and in the original writings of some of the leading Stoic thinkers, such as Epictetus, Seneca, and Marcus Aurelius.

Stoicism is often misunderstood as being an emotionless philosophy, but it is actually the opposite. The main intention is to help us lead our best, happiest, most fulfilling lives. Perhaps the most important virtue to Stoics is courage, which is as important today as it was in ancient times.

In a certain way, Stoics actually relish the challenge of unfortunate events, because they offer a chance for us to see what we are made of. Somewhere around 50 CE, Seneca wrote that "if you have passed through life without an opponent, no one can ever know what you are capable of, not even you."

If courage (in the face of unfortunate events) is the most important Stoic virtue, then the most important practice in Stoic philosophy is differentiating between what we have control over (and thus can influence) and what we don't have control over (and thus shouldn't worry about). It is important to make this a daily practice—always asking yourself what aspects of a given situation are within or outside of your control.

What matters most to a Stoic is not the situation that they find themselves in (which is often not in your control), nor is it their initial immediate reaction (which in many cases is purely biological, such as a stress response), but rather it is how they *respond* to the situation (which is entirely in your control). Your response to a given situation is what really matters, because it is what you can manage. For example, let's say you get fired from your job because of a difference of opinion with your boss. Your first *reaction* might be anger, but it is your *response after that reaction* that matters most to your ability to resolve the situation and move forward. Likewise, we might have an initial feeling of panic if the stock market crashes (this is simply a natural physiological fight-or-flight reaction), but our response that comes next is what really matters (in fact, it is the only thing that matters).

Think about the people who are routinely put in some of the most stressful situations, such as soldiers and first responders. They are not necessarily braver than other people, but they are definitely better prepared to respond to a stressful situation because of their training. In a similar fashion, we can train our emotional response muscles to help us move beyond initial reaction to appropriate response. Epictetus wrote, "Every event has two handles, one by which it can be carried, and one by which it can't. If your brother does you wrong, don't grab it by his wronging, because this is the handle incapable of lifting it. Instead, use the other—that he is your brother, that you were raised together, and then you will have hold of the handle that carries."

Our family motto since our kids were very young has been, "The only difference between an ordeal and an adventure is attitude." This pithy blurb—variously attributed to many people and nobody—succinctly sums up the philosophy that we try to (mostly) live by. We do our very best to have a mindset of asking "Do I have control over this?" followed by an actset of "Yes, and." This helps put us in motion toward improving what we can and not worrying about the rest.

What Are Emotions Anyway?

None of us could go through life without experiencing emotions—nor would we want to. Emotions, as messy as they can be, help us to survive and thrive. Fear helps alert us to threats. Love promotes social bonds. Joy moves us toward things that make us feel good. Hope encourages us to plan for the future. Even the range of challenging emotions that make us feel bad in certain ways, such as anger, irritation, and sadness, have value in helping us navigate and make sense of the complex social world in which we live.

Emotions are wonderfully and frustratingly complex, operating on multiple conscious and subconscious levels simultaneously. Our head brains are in a constant state of receiving informative signals from inside and outside the body. Some of these signals come from our lower, primitive brain, which may be more attuned to sensing fear and potential threats at a subconscious level, and then they travel upward to our more modern, reasoning brain (the frontal cortex). Other signals may be generated directly in our prefrontal cortex based on our experiences, learning, memories, and cultural context. Still other signals that eventually become distilled into emotions come from our gut brain, heart brain, immune axis, external environment, physical surroundings, and many other inputs.

As discussed earlier, the idea that creative people are "right-brained" while analytical people are "left-brained" is overly simplistic. Newer ideas about our complex emotions describe how our brain uses its most advanced and distinctly human prefrontal cortex to integrate signals coming from myriad internal and external sources to construct emotions on demand in relation to each and every unique situation.

In addition, we know that more than half of our emotional vocabulary occurs outside of our brain—through our facial expressions, body posture, and touching, but also through body sensations, such as our heart rate, breathing patterns, muscle tension, nerve tingles, and so many others. It is a wonder that even our highly evolved human brains can integrate all these signals into a coherent emotional tapestry—and most of the time (though not always), we do just fine. So while many emotional signals very well might emanate from bottom/top/left/right/internal/external portions of our brain, it's actually the *integration* of all these signals across a vast interacting neural network that enables us to label and regulate any particular feeling.

Sometimes we get into trouble when these myriad signals get mixed up or get stuck in a loop, such as when a simple stressor becomes chronic and we spiral to anxiety, depression, and burnout. This is where the difference between a short-term emotion (which tends to be more of a front-and-center feeling) and a longer-term mood (which tends to be in the background of our consciousness) can become an important distinction. As we discussed earlier about our head brain, whether we are talking about the lower subcortex, with the primitive amygdala (fear), hippocampus (memory), and hypothalamus (stress), or the upper prefrontal cortex, with advanced and complex emotional tasks of labeling, identifying, and responding to our emotions, it is important to reemphasize that our brain is always working as a coordinated system (called a *neural network*) rather than as isolated sections. This is important because this network can also adapt and change both its function and its structure based on its activity. Neurons that fire together, as they say, wire together. This means that we can stimulate the growth of new neuronal pathways with consistent thought patterns. These neurogenic patterns can be positive, such as a feeling of novelty that can be generated by learning or traveling, or they can be negative, such as with stress or sleep loss that are known to slow neurogenesis. In response to consistent activation of neural firing patterns, specialized areas of the brain such as the amygdala can become more or less reactive to fear, the hypothalamus can become more or less responsive to stress, and the hippocampus can become more or less able to retain and retrieve memories. It's encouraging to note that we actually have a great deal of control over the ways these neural networks develop over time. For example, we know that chronic stress can slow down the process of neurogenesis, whereas exercise and novelty (such as traveling to new places and learning new things) can accelerate neurogenesis—even well into old age.

The best news of all about our complex network of feelings is that scientists consider emotions and moods to be mostly under our control to modulate in a positive direction because only a small portion is due to genetics or heritability (around 30 percent), while the rest comes from our environmental influences, including social connections and lifestyle factors such as patterns of diet, exercise, and sleep.

Emotional Regulation

Our ability to acknowledge, share, and manage our emotions is directly related to our overall level of happiness and mental fitness. A lot of this ability to manage our emotions occurs in the reasoning section of our head brain, the prefrontal cortex. But this area is strongly affected by stress, blood sugar levels, lack of sleep, depression, and anxiety. This is why we often make bad choices when we're tired or hungry or stressed out and have trouble making any decisions at all when we're depressed or anxious.

Because our prefrontal cortex is so important for emotional regulation, and because it can get hijacked by our stressful world, we need a strategy that helps us *respond* rather than merely *react* to powerful emotions. I use a simple three-step technique that can help with reappraisal of an emotionally charged situation. I call it the *frame it, name it, tame it* approach, and it works like this:

Frame it.

Let's say another driver cuts you off in traffic or your boss makes a dismissive comment about one of your ideas. Your initial reaction might be a flash of anger at the other driver or animosity toward your boss, but we can reframe those feelings. You might think to yourself that the reason the other driver cut you off is that they're rushing to their daughter's soccer practice or to an important job interview. You might imagine that your boss was curt and dismissive because she is stressed about the current sales numbers and just lacks the bandwidth to see the brilliance of your proposal. We don't want to ignore or suppress our feelings, but we can use our abilities for empathy and compassion to see the situation from the other person's perspective so we can frame the situation in a way that minimizes its emotional impact.

Name it.

We don't want to ignore or suppress our emotions. Rather, we want to acknowledge what we are feeling as precisely as possible using our emotional vocabulary. Are we feeling stress or irritation or sadness or envy or fear or any of dozens of other emotions? The more specific and granular you can get, the better. When we can name the emotion, by acknowledging not just the situation but precisely how the situation makes us *feel*, then we can pinpoint the best way to cope.

Tame it.

When we know what emotion we are dealing with, we can manage it in an appropriate way. For example, if you are often irritated around your wealthy friend, you might find that your discomfort is actually envy or spite or disappointment—and each of these reactions can benefit from a slightly different solution. Many times, you will find that by simply reframing the situation and naming how it makes you feel, you are already in a more mindful and aware state that enables you to practice acceptance and nonreactivity to even the most emotionally charged situations. Reframing the situation of being uncomfortable hearing about your wealthy friend's big house, expensive car, or exotic vacation (maybe he is bragging to appear successful in one area because he feels insecure about some other aspect of his life) and naming the envy that you feel because your friend has something that you also want enables you to move toward a solution. You might start saving more money or earning more through a side gig to get the house or car you desire or even volunteering to do charity work abroad so you can travel. Or you might start focusing yourself more toward areas where you are successful in your own life.

Whatever the eventual solution, you can use these three simple steps—*frame it, name it, tame it*—to move yourself from irritation to envy to hope instead of just being stuck.

Positive Emotions

Emotions such as happiness, joy, contentment, love, compassion, and gratitude are much more than simply good feelings. The more we experience these positive emotions, the more likely we are to expand our creativity, connect with others, and seek out opportunities (sometimes referred to as the *broaden and build* theory of human development). Numerous research studies have shown that people who experience positive emotions have superior physical health. They have fewer heart attacks and strokes, stronger immune systems, and lower stress hormones, and they live longer. But they also have superior mental fitness, with lower incidence of depression and anxiety and a heightened ability to buffer distress and remain resilient when the stuff hits the fan.

This ability to be resilient in the face of different stressors can be thought of somewhat like a psychological immune system, where positive emotions don't just shield us from mental and physical health problems, but they also improve our ability to turn a bad situation into a better one by encouraging us to engage in the very behaviors that feed positive emotions. This can quite directly change a negative downward spiral such as depression or burnout into a positive upward spiral toward better psychological vigor. Our thoughts and behaviors can reverse a vicious negative cycle of feeling worse and worse and turn it into a virtuous positive cycle of feeling better and better—sort of like a happy snowball effect where positive emotions don't only *emerge* from strong relationships and good health, but they *promote* them.

It is important to understand that our brains are actually wired to be more attuned to negative experiences than to positive ones. This negativity bias is why we can feel terrible after hearing a dozen compliments or getting numerous likes and then a single complaint or rejection. Some studies have shown that we need three positive experiences to counteract each negative emotion—and that is just to keep us in a neutral emotional state. One very effective technique to improve our emotional state is to create a daily diet of happy microemotions by using mindfulness techniques and gratitude moments sprinkled throughout the day to continuously buffer the negative emotions that come at us on a regular basis. (I personally use the reminders to stand and breathe that my Apple Watch sends me throughout the day to quietly express gratitude for little things, such as the cup of coffee I might be enjoying, the sunny day, or my goofy dog.)

The idea of fostering positive emotions to improve mental fitness and physical health does not mean that we simply ignore negative thoughts or gloss over difficulties by just thinking happy thoughts. However, there are a number of simple approaches to get our thoughts moving in the right direction, from exercise (which bathes your body and brain in feel-good neurotransmitters) to interacting with strangers (hold the door or say good morning—even small interactions can boost mood). What you might find is that thoughts often follow behaviors. Even if you don't feel like doing something, just doing it can help the feeling follow. Just getting started can often help you feel like continuing.

Some studies have suggested that we're happiest in our twenties (when we're young and healthy and optimistic about our future) and most unhappy in our thirties (due to the stress of raising kids and early careers) and forties (due to the stress of mid-careers and finances).

Typically, we reach our lowest happiness levels around the age of fifty. But the good news is that happiness levels tend to rise again after the age of fifty—possibly because the kids are out on their own or because we've settled into a career rhythm (and hopefully have not just settled with our lot in life), or perhaps we've finally learned to cope better with stress. Even better news is that we can use many of the tools from positive psychology and nutritional psychology to feed the right information to our minds and bodies.

What Makes Us Happy?

So what actually makes us happy? You have undoubtedly heard the old saying "Money doesn't buy happiness." But it actually *does*—at least to a point. After meeting your basics needs for food, shelter, and safety, happiness increases with wealth up to about $70,000 per year, and then it completely levels off. Numerous studies have shown this leveling-off effect of wealth on happiness, and yet financial stress is by far the leading source of psychological stress in national surveys year in and year out. The stress of making ends meet, the economy, job security, and the general balancing of needs versus wants greets us in the morning and puts us to bed at night.

It might to surprise you, however, that if you peel back the layers of what actually is stressing people out, it is not the money per se but what the money provides in terms of feelings of self-worth (and comparison to others) and especially of autonomy. A greater financial reservoir allows us to make choices that we otherwise could not make. It replaces a certain level of financial stress with financial freedom. Money doesn't *directly* buy happiness, but struggling financially can certainly limit our time, opportunities, and day-to-day enjoyment. It can limit our ability to dream about and plan for the future, and the chronic stress that comes from financial worries can lead to a drip-by-drip erosion of our mental fitness.

When people talk about having financial freedom, they are referring to the fact that having enough money permits us the chance to make our own choices. This is what psychology researchers refer to as *autonomy*:

the ability to have a say in what we do, when we do it, how we do it, and who we do it with.

The secret to happiness is freedom, and the secret to freedom is courage.
— Thucydides

There is no shortage of pithy articles and lists all over the internet promising things like the "top five ways to boost your happiness." Some of these simple tips can actually be quite beneficial, such as helping us understand that experiences are more strongly associated with boosts in happiness than belongings are. So taking an epic trip might make you happier for longer than buying a new car. Likewise, relationships and work satisfaction are stronger predictors of happiness and even better at predicting fulfillment (a profound sense of satisfaction) that provides a deeper meaning to your everyday actions and a longer-lasting feeling of well-being. It is important to note that while some of these simple tips might help us feel slightly better temporarily, research studies show us that three factors emerge over and over again in being key determinants of our long-term happiness and resilience:

➤ Autonomy—being able to make your own choices and decisions versus having them imposed on you

➤ Mastery—being good at something but also using that expertise to assist others

➤ Purpose—feeling that what you do matters to others, whether that is just one other person, your family, your coworkers, or your community or a greater mission outside of yourself

People who find a way to combine autonomy, mastery, and purpose (AMP) emerge in these studies as having the highest happiness scores on a day-to-day basis and also rank as the most resilient to future episodes of anxiety, depression, or burnout.

Martin Seligman, who is often held up as the father of positive psychology, posits a similar theory of authentic happiness, which identifies five components (PERMA) that are very much in alignment with the core AMP factors:

> Positive emotion—such as hope, contentment, and gratitude

> Engagement—being completely immersed in an enjoyable activity you're skilled at, like work or a sport or hobby (losing yourself in flow)

> Relationships—with individuals or groups that provide a supportive connection and nurturing environment

> Meaning—feeling that you are part of a bigger mission

> Accomplishments—pursuing and reaching goals that are meaningful to you

What Makes Us *Un*happy?

Nobody wants to experience distressing emotions such as fear, anger, sadness, anxiety, and shame. But paying attention to them and acknowledging them rather than suppressing them can help us prioritize and prepare for action. Studies have shown that people with higher levels of unmanaged anger often have a greater degree of relationship strife and experience worse cardiovascular health as well as higher rates of obesity, diabetes, insomnia, immune problems, migraines, depression, and drug and alcohol addiction.

On the other hand, studies have also shown that people who accept negative emotions, versus ignoring them or pushing them away, tend to experience less depression and anxiety and greater mental fitness and physical well-being. Distressing emotions such as anger, fear, and shame are best experienced as moderating emotions. We want enough distress to help clarify our thinking and motivate our actions but not so much that we're debilitated by it. Fear is an interesting example. Millions of people like to go to scary movies or participate in exhilarating hobbies such as skydiving or rock climbing—seeking out fear. We routinely use fear to inject a jolt of spice into our lives, but we wouldn't want to experience those same feelings of fear if we're putting our kids to bed or trying to relax with a good book.

While fear tends to be focused on a specific external thing that is present and could possibly cause you harm, the related emotion of anxiety is nonspecific and internal and often caused by an imagined and possibly unlikely threat. Anxiety can be much more difficult to deal with because you often can't accurately describe what it is that is causing you to feel unsettled or why; you can't quite put your finger on it. You might be interested to know that threats to our social identity, including threats to self-worth and feelings of envy and insecurity, have been shown to produce the most dramatic spikes in feelings of stress and anxiety. In the same Goldilocks scenario with other distressing emotions, a little bit of anxiety can help motivate us to get our ducks in a row, but too much interferes with our ability to focus on other important issues in our life.

Sadness and depression are among the most common of the distressing negative emotions, but the two are not the same. Sadness is an emotion marked by feelings of loss and helplessness, while depression goes beyond merely being a prolonged state of sadness to include feelings of hopelessness, guilt, low self-worth, brain fog, sleep problems, fatigue, and lack of joy and pleasure (even for events and activities that previously provided enjoyment). It's not possible to just snap yourself out of either sadness or depression—a common myth—but it is very possible to work your way through them by using these feelings as potent social-bonding opportunities. For example, if you are feeling sad or depressed, asking someone else for help (even if you don't feel like doing so) can spark the social connection that can often stop depression in its tracks. Similarly, when we are feeling fine, we can use empathy to rally around another person facing difficulty—simultaneously helping them and helping ourselves.

The ability to feel sadness appropriately is a mark of emotional health. We want to feel those emotions as we use lifestyle approaches such as diet, exercise, sleep, and mindfulness to improve how we feel. Medications such as antidepressants and antianxiety drugs might be somewhat helpful in suppressing our ability to feel *any* emotions—negative and positive—so we might feel less bad temporarily, but we certainly don't feel good when using these drugs. Many antidepressant users report not being able to feel much of anything; they just feel sort of flat, so life loses a lot of its color and excitement. In fact, newer research has suggested that much of the improvement in depression indices with antidepressant drugs is a placebo effect (which works in about half of the people who try them), but the longer-term side effects—including weight gain, fatigue, loss of libido, and severe withdrawal symptoms when you try to quit—make these drugs something you would want to consider only as a last resort.

All of these negative distressing emotions respond positively to lifestyle interventions, such as cognitive behavioral therapy, mindfulness techniques like reframing and gratitude, deep breathing, and other approaches that we can use to feed our minds the most nourishing signals. Just as consuming the right diet of nutrients keeps our gut healthy and consuming the right diet of physical activity keeps our heart healthy, consuming the right diet of thoughts into our brain on a regular basis keeps us mentally fit with a strong emotional regulation system.

When Feelings Become Physical

There is a direct link between the mental pain of stress, depression, anxiety, and burnout, and physical pain, such as back pain, neck pain, stomachaches, migraines, fibromyalgia, and others. Somatization is when emotional concerns are experienced as physical symptoms. But the direction can go both ways, with physical pain, especially when it is chronic, leading to emotional distress.

This makes sense physiologically and biochemically, because a lot of the neurological pathways in the brain for pain and emotion are shared regions, and the same excessive inflammatory signals have been identified in mental conditions (depression) and physical conditions (heart disease and arthritis). A potential silver lining here is that numerous nondrug interventions such as positive emotions, deep breathing, pleasant smells (essential oils), physical touch (massage), and motivating music can help block pain signals as effectively as pain medications.

Emotions of Wonder

Humans are hardwired to seek out interesting experiences to satisfy our curiosity and to get that sensation of wow and wonder that helps us broaden our horizons. These emotions encourage us to explore, learn, solve problems, generate ideas, and connect with others. Exposing ourselves regularly to wonder can also be a pathway to ease distress and enhance mental fitness. Research has shown that wonder can reduce activity in the brain's default mode network, calming the self-focused chattering that often dominates our thoughts, especially when we are under stress. Feelings of amusement, interest, and especially awe (all of which generate dopamine production to motivate us) can enable us to become fully absorbed and immersed in something to the degree that our perspective shifts away from ourselves and outward toward wonder, helping us achieve a Zen-like state similar to what comes through meditation. People who are more open as a personality trait tend to also be more curious and express a higher degree of interest about the world around them and thus tend to be predisposed to experiencing positive emotions of wonder.

Even though I use a variety of mindfulness techniques such as deep breathing and expressing gratitude to help calm my own stress responses, formal practices of meditation or yoga are not really my cup of tea (despite the fact that I'm well aware of the scientific evidence for their effectiveness). Formal meditation and yoga practice might be wonderful for lots of people (and you really should give them a try to see for yourself), but I've found that what works best for me personally is what I call *moving meditation*. It generally involves running or cycling long distances and putting myself as often as possible in or near awe-inducing natural settings such as mountains, valleys, deserts, oceans, rivers, and other places where the vastness of nature can blow my mind.

One of the really interesting aspects of experiencing awe is that it fosters feelings of connection to others (even when you might be by yourself on an isolated mountainside) and of kindness and generosity—possibly because the experience of awe diminishes the self-focused ego and allows for focus on group well-being. Research has shown that awe is the most strongly linked of all the positive emotions to increases in dopamine (motivation) and oxytocin (connection) as well as to reductions in cortisol (stress) and inflammatory cytokines (depression). It might be this combination of changes in the brain's electrical activity and biochemical balance that enables the euphoric sensations of feeling at one with others and with the universe, and we can readily achieve it through a variety of approaches, from spiritual experiences such as prayer to secular practices such as meditation and physical movement meditations such as exercise (especially outside).

Social Connections and the Loneliness Epidemic

The Harvard Study of Adult Development, sometimes referred to as the Harvard Longevity Study, has been running for more than seventy-five years. It has shown quite convincingly that the best predictor of a long and happy life is the strength of our relationships. Humans are hardwired for social connection. It lowers cortisol (stress) and increases both dopamine (motivation) and oxytocin (bonding), but only when those social connections are supportive. If your social engagements are negative or tense, they can actually lead away from happiness and toward not only unhappiness but to health problems such as obesity, diabetes, and addictive behaviors (which means you should either ditch your negative friends for some positive ones or see if you can get those pessimists to move with you toward a more optimistic future).

Perhaps the strongest social connection of all is love, and the most enduring forms of love are equal parts desire (testosterone), passion (dopamine), and attachment (oxytocin). Gratitude runs a close second, because it is one of the positive emotions that is not only strongly linked to better health but also easily engaged by simple thoughts or more formal approaches such as keeping a gratitude journal. Hope is another emotion that can be engaged at will. Hope is sometimes more specifically defined as an attitude rather than as an emotion, but we will consider it as an emotion for our purposes of boosting mental fitness because fostering hope is so effective for buffering the detrimental effects of chronic stress. Like optimism, hope has been linked to higher levels of happiness, resilience, mental fitness, and physical health. In fact, hope can be every bit as potent as any medication—it can boost mood, quell pain, and directly enhance our body's ability to heal. In order to engage hope on demand to motivate our forward progress, we need to cultivate three factors that link directly back to the key factors associated with overall happiness and resilience:

➤ A sense of control—knowing that we can affect our fate in a positive direction

➤ Belief in the value of something important enough to work toward

➤ Community—being part of a group that values the same things we do

Empathy is the ability to imagine and feel another person's emotions—to put yourself in their shoes. Feelings of empathy are thought to be due, at least in part, to the actions of specialized mirror neurons in the brain that allow us to feel an emotion when we watch someone else having that emotion. Compassion, which is related to empathy, is a social emotion felt in response to another person's suffering, but which is also linked to feelings of caring and wanting to relieve the suffering. Some research suggests that compassion is healthier than mere empathy because of the greater affiliation and positive emotion that comes from wanting to help someone else (and the surge of calming oxytocin). Helping others can help you—even if you are just *thinking* about helping them and genuinely wanting good things to come their way.

One way to cultivate your own compassion is with a simple form of meditation known as loving-kindness meditation, which simply involves focusing on another person (a loved one, a stranger, even an enemy) and feeling compassion for that person's suffering. You might think of this as being virtually connected to others. Some practitioners of loving-kindness meditation will combine these thoughts with deep breathing while they generate, send out, and reflect on the warm feelings of these wishes, such as the following:

➤ May x be safe.

➤ May x be healthy.

➤ May x be happy.

If you are religious, the idea of loving-kindness meditation will look familiar. It is very much the secular version of saying a prayer for someone or lighting a candle in the Catholic tradition or focusing energy in a variety of Eastern traditions. They all share the common factors of calm, focused compassion that helps bolster our mental fitness.

What Is the Right Diet to Nourish Your Brain?

If you are nourishing your brain with a steady diet of political yelling on the nightly news or whatever nonsense YouTube's algorithm decides to serve up, then your mental fitness might be in the same shape as a body built on junk food.

The concept of self-improvement is very trendy. People love the *idea* of improving themselves with a sharper mind, a sleeker body, and a more open and expansive mindset. But the dirty little secret of actually getting better and becoming the best version of your future self is that it can be hard work!

We can't just *think about* getting better; we have to *do* it. We have to *practice* it every day. We have to embrace the process and love the journey every bit as much as we love the idea of reaching our destination of better (which, if we are doing it right, we will never quite achieve). If we can do that by consistently integrating a few improvement practices into our hectic lives, then we can improve our mental fitness step-by-step, helping catapult us toward becoming our best selves.

Here is a simple checklist of some of my favorite (and most effective) steps to help us regulate our emotions, strengthen our mindset, and bolster our mental fitness. Keep in mind that "simple" does not always mean "easy," but these steps will work for you if you work with them.

✓ MENTAL FITNESS CHECKLIST

❑ The 3 Cs

In any given stressful situation, pause for a moment and ask yourself three key questions—what I call the 3 Cs:

➤ What can I control?

➤ Who can I connect with?

➤ How can I contribute (either to a cause or to a project that helps someone else solve their problems)?

❑ Use positive self-talk and optimism.

Positive self-talk and optimism are combined for a common technique that has helped prisoners of war and people dealing with trauma, abuse, and medical problems keep going. Stay calm, and focus on what you can control. Start with the good, and stay realistic about the situation. Do one little thing to make it a bit better, then another little thing and another, cascading upward positivity as opposed to spiraling downward negativity. Olympic athletes use positive self-talk to help them focus on now, which is really the only thing that matters when you either need to do your best or just get through this moment.

☐ Move!

The most resilient people have a regular exercise habit. The mild to moderate stress of exercise trains us to adapt to the bigger and more important stressors of life's challenges. Stressing our body (and mind) a little bit every day helps us to handle the big stresses that will inevitably come.

☐ Play the game.

The best way to deal with stress is to see problems as challenges rather than as threats. Stop seeing your problems as irritating inconveniences and more as interesting challenges to be overcome as if you were playing a video game or board game. Give yourself rewards for unlocking the next achievement and advancing to the next round.

☐ Laugh.

Laugh—at both yourself and at what you're doing and at the situation in general. Humor (in the right amounts, balanced with seriousness) can be used to reduce the threatening nature of a stressful situation.

☐ Find purpose and meaning.

The number one thing that stands out among people who triumph over tragedy is that they have identified a greater purpose or some form of meaning in life. This can be a religious belief or simply a form of deep connection with others or conviction in a movement (the word *religion* comes from the Latin *religare*, meaning "to bind," so the concept of religion is as much about being connected to a community as it is about belief in any deity). This goes hand in hand with a tendency toward altruism and selflessness—the ability to have concern for the well-being of others without any expectation of a direct benefit to yourself. Being part of a community of like-minded individuals working together toward a common purpose can help to strengthen your resolve, especially in the face of stressful events and adversity. Helping others is an effective way to take you out of yourself. It helps you rise above your own concerns and fears about the situation and moves you from being a victim toward being a helper or a rescuer. When others look to you for skill and leadership, it raises their confidence as well as your confidence that we will all get through the situation together.

☐ Label your stresses.

Use the *frame it, name it, tame it* approach described earlier to help reappraise negative situations and move them toward positive action.

☐ Savor beauty.

Actively put yourself in situations where you can feel awe on a daily basis, even if it is just a mindful walk outside where you can look at the sky, clouds, sun, or stars.

☐ Breathe!

Breathing might just be the easiest thing that most of us do all wrong, and that can be a huge mistake. Our nasal cavity is a direct line to our brain's emotional and memory centers (via sensory neurons that link to the olfactory bulb). This is why a familiar scent can bring on a wave of memories and why we can use techniques such as aromatherapy to treat stress and anxiety with near-immediate effects. Because these neurons sense the passage of air in and out of the nasal cavity, we can use breathing techniques to synchronize brain waves to the rhythm of our breath. For example, deep rhythmic breathing in and out through our nose can stimulate the vagus nerve that runs the entire length of our gut-heart-brain axis to reduce stress, slow our heart rate, and reduce blood pressure (five to six breaths per minute). If you want to be a little more advanced, deep and slow nasal breathing at a rate of only three breaths per minute can shift the brain toward production of more of the brain-repairing theta waves that dominate deep phases of sleep (this is why super slow and deep breathing is so effective for helping us fall asleep at night). Another breathing technique that is extremely effective in counteracting stress, anxiety, and panic attacks is to perform two large inhalations followed by a hold and a long, slow exhalation. This technique fills your lungs on the first inhalation and then overfills your lungs on the second inhalation, and the entire process activates a profound and immediate calming response via your vagus nerve and PNS.

☐ Slow down—especially when eating.

This is one that I am often guilty of not adhering to very well. I am often impatient, in a rush, and hurrying to finish one thing and move on to the next thing. Hey, nobody is perfect, but I am trying! Growing research around mindful eating is showing that becoming more aware of our food—not just how it tastes, but noticing and appreciating the various smells, textures, colors, and temperatures—can improve digestion, appetite control, blood sugar balance, and weight management. Enjoying a meal with others also brings in a social element that improves a variety of mental fitness parameters, such as satisfaction, enjoyment, connection, and contentedness.

☐ Cultivate hope.

Cultivate hope by imagining your best self on the other side of a challenge. Visualize how a neutral third-party might view your situation or how you will feel about this a month from now.

☐ Express gratitude.

Express gratitude even for the smallest things.

☐ Practice loving-kindness meditation.

Practice loving-kindness meditation by sending good vibes out to others and into the universe in general.

☐ Connect.

Connect with others, and do something to help them (which helps you).

☐ Cultivate a beginner's mind.

Learn something new. Even though you absolutely want to work toward achieving mastery in certain areas, you can't know everything or always be the best at everything. Maintaining an attitude of enthusiastic and open curiosity and the willingness to avoid falling into preconceived notions based on past experiences can often feel uncomfortable but can also feel exhilarating if approached with the right frame of mind.

You can't stop the hurricane, but you can be the tree that bends with the wind and snaps back up. Using some of these techniques can help us to be flexible and enable us to develop and maintain the mindset that leads to the resilience and mental fitness that we need to keep going (and even become better) when times get difficult.

CHAPTER 9

DIETARY SUPPLEMENTS

In my very first book, *The Cortisol Connection* (2002), I wrote about how chronic stress can "make you fat and ruin your health," and I offered a number of natural lifestyle approaches to help readers reduce their stress, control their cortisol, and improve their mental and physical health. In that first book, I had a plan that I called the "SENSE" program, with each letter representing one of the main concepts:

S = stress/sleep management

E = exercise

N = nutrition

S = supplements

E = evaluation

Nearly twenty years later, the steps in SENSE remain effective approaches to improving mental and physical health (updated to reflect advances in science, such as our understanding of the microbiome and the gut-heart-brain axis).

These days, however, whenever I educate people about SENSE, I flip the *S*'s so "supplements" becomes the first *S* and the first step of the program. This is not because supplements are more important than any of the other steps, nor is it because supplements can replace any other aspect of SENSE, but rather because they can be a heck of a lot easier for a lot of people to integrate into their busy, stressful, modern lives. What I have found over the last two decades of research is that properly formulated dietary supplements can help to reduce stress and stress-eating enough for someone to start making better choices about their daily diet. They can help to reduce fatigue and boost energy levels enough for someone to finally feel like becoming physically active. They can reduce tension and anxiety enough for someone to relax and get a good night's sleep with ample time in REM and deep sleep. In short, supplements can facilitate the adoption of the healthy lifestyle behaviors that we all know we need to do in the first place but that we often do not do because we are too tired, stressed, or depressed. We have seen this "supplements can help us make better choices" phenomenon over and over in research studies and in community lifestyle programs, and as long as we keep in mind that supplements are part of the overall program—and not the entire program—we have the correct approach to make meaningful strides toward better mental fitness.

I have written two award-winning academic textbooks on dietary supplements, but rather than write an exhaustive encyclopedia of all the possible vitamins, minerals, herbals, amino acids, plant extracts, and all manner of exotic natural medicines from around the world, I intend this chapter to be more of a "best of" overview of supplements that can be particularly effective for improving mental fitness by optimizing signaling across the entire gut-heart-brain axis.

Each supplement is described in terms of the scientific and medical evidence for its effects on mental fitness. The four sections to follow are divided into our three "brains" (gut brain, head brain, and heart brain) and their connecting axis (immune system, endocrine system, endocannabinoid system, nervous system, etc.). Keep in mind, however, that this separation is somewhat artificial because, for example, while a specific strain of probiotic bacteria might "work in the gut" and thus be included in the "gut brain" section, it very likely is exerting its benefits to reduce depression and improve mood at the level of the "head brain."

In contrast to synthetic prescription pharmaceuticals and even over-the-counter drugs, dietary supplements are extremely safe, with adverse events or side effects being exceedingly rare. That said, they do happen from time to time, and they are almost impossible to predict because of differences between product formulations, personal health status, individual medication regimens, and numerous lifestyle factors (diet, sleep, stress, and more). Any individual who is under medical supervision for a chronic disease or who is taking prescription or over-the-counter medications should always check with their health-care provider before adding any dietary supplement to their daily regimen. Likewise, women should understand that any dietary supplement that they are considering taking is unlikely to have been specifically researched or found to be safe under conditions of pregnancy or lactation, so it is best to avoid "herbal medicine" types of supplements during these higher risk times of life (but there are often suitable food-based alternatives that can be substituted as needed to maintain mental fitness for new and expecting moms).

Supplements to Support the Gut Brain

As we discussed in chapter 2, the gut, as our "second brain," is involved in a great deal more than simply digestion of food and absorption of nutrients. Having optimal gut function supports immune function, inflammatory balance, and mental fitness. Here are my top recommendations for supplements to support our gut brain.

Probiotics

Probiotics are defined by the International Scientific Association for Probiotics and Prebiotics (ISAPP) as "live microorganisms that, when administered in adequate amounts, confer a health benefit on the host." The word *probiotic* means "promoting life" and is derived from the Greek *pro*, indicating "promoting," and *biotic*, indicating "life." The original discovery of probiotics by eventual Nobel Prize–winning scientist Élie Metchnikoff came about one hundred years ago when he observed how rural Bulgarian farmers maintained health, resisted illness, and lived to very old ages despite extreme poverty and difficult lives. He theorized that the sour/fermented milk that constituted an important part of their diet was responsible for their health.

Probiotic research has come a long way since Dr. Metchnikoff's days. Now we still recommend fermented foods like yogurt, kombucha, and kimchi (which all contain various mixtures of probiotic bacteria) for general health benefits, but we can also recommend specific probiotic strains for targeted benefits. For example, the emerging field of nutritional psychology shows us a range of clinically validated probiotic strains that are able to improve mood and well-being and reduce depression and anxiety indexes. Three of the best-supported strains for mental fitness in humans are *Lactobacillus helveticus* R0052, *Bifidobacterium longum* R0175, and *Lactobacillus rhamnosus* R0011.

Lactobacillus helveticus R0052 decreases neuroinflammation, improves serotonin metabolism, decreases anxiety, restores cognitive function, reduces inflammation, mediates serotonergic transmission, and elicits antianxiety and antidepressant responses.

Bifidobacterium longum R0175 decreases stress response, facilitates antidepressant responses, decreases anxiety, and enhances cognitive function.

Lactobacillus rhamnosus R0011 reduces anxiety and depression and improves GABA neurotransmission (the body's primary relaxing neurotransmitter).

Just a quick word about the strain-specific benefits of probiotics. Most commercial products do not indicate which strain is contained in the supplement. If you don't know the strain, then you really have no idea of the benefit (if any) that the product is supposed to be delivering. For example, *Lactobacillus* (genus) *rhamnosus* (species) R0011 (strain) is effective for reducing anxiety and depression, while another *Lactobacillus rhamnosus* strain (GG) is great for traveler's diarrhea, another (LR-32) is good for constipation, and yet another (GR-1) can treat and prevent yeast infections. As you can imagine, seeing only "*Lactobacillus rhamnosus*" (genus/species) on the label of a product does not tell you very much and certainly does not let you know what to expect from a given product. You need to know the strain and know that the strain has been clinically validated in humans for the specific benefit you're looking for.

Prebiotics

Prebiotics are defined by the ISAPP as "a substrate that is selectively utilized by host microorganisms conferring a health benefit," which means that prebiotics can "feed and support" the health and function of probiotic bacteria. Prebiotics are frequently equated with dietary fibers, but only a subset of dietary fibers actually qualify as prebiotics. According to the broad scientific definition, prebiotics need not be forms of dietary fiber at all, so plant extracts such as polyphenols/flavonoids and yeast/mushroom glucans can induce a prebiotic effect by helping support the function of probiotic bacteria in the gut. Prebiotics should also preferentially and selectively support the growth of beneficial bacteria families, such as *Lactobacillus, Bifidobacterium, Akkermansia*—and not support the growth of detrimental bacterial species. Here are some of the best-supported prebiotics:

Galacto-oligosaccharides belong to a special group of nutrient fibers called oligosaccharides that naturally feed and stimulate the growth of preferred bacteria in the gut. It resets and increases friendly gut bacteria, maintains immune health, and works in your gut to support your natural microbiome balance. It's a highly effective and natural way of increasing the preferred bacteria in your gut to both control inflammation and support mental fitness.

Isomalto-oligosaccharides are a special combination of naturally occurring plant fibers that are clinically shown to improve the growth of "good" gut bacteria. They act as a specific prebiotic that feeds the probiotic genus *Lactobacillus* and *Bifidobacterium* and stimulates production of short-chain fatty acids.

Galactomannan, also known as PHGG (partially hydrolyzed guar gum), is sourced from the guar bean, a clinically proven prebiotic fiber that helps improve growth and viability of beneficial bacteria within the intestinal tract, including *Bifidobacterium* and *Lactobacillus*. PHGG ferments very slowly, so there's significantly less gas and bloating compared to many other types of fermentable fiber (the fermentation indicates that our gut bacteria are digesting this fiber as a fuel source).

Acacia gum is also referred to as "gum arabic" and is derived from the natural sap of the acacia tree that grows natively in parts of Africa, Pakistan, and India. The sap/gum is dried and crushed into a fine powder that is rich in prebiotic fibers that support the growth and metabolism of "good" bacteria in our gut. In several studies, acacia gum was shown to produce a greater increase in *Bifidobacterium* and *Lactobacillus* than an equal dose of inulin (another prebiotic fiber, often extracted from chicory) and resulted in fewer gastrointestinal side effects, such as gas and bloating.

One factor that I particularly like about each of these prebiotic fibers is that they do not "just" support the growth of beneficial bacteria and promote gut integrity, but they also have direct benefits for important aspects of mental fitness. For example, acacia gum is routinely claimed to simply help people "feel better," and specific anti-stress and mood-boosting effects are under study right now. Both GOS and galactomannan have previously been shown to improve stress resilience (in healthy stressed adults) and improve stress, irritability, and behavior in autistic children. Think about that for a moment—that a "fiber" can help to improve behavior in kids with autism, which is a notoriously hard-to-manage collection of dysfunctions across the entire gut-brain axis. The clinical studies in this area are in agreement that the prebiotic fiber is having a consistent metabolic effect at the level of the microbiome (increased production of neurotransmitters and short-chain fatty acids), which have beneficial signaling effects across the nervous system and immune system, reaching the brain where tension and irritability are reduced and calmness and focus are enhanced. These early findings are potentially revolutionary—and not just for anyone struggling with autism (including their caregivers), but for anyone who wants to reach the peak of their own mental fitness potential.

Postbiotics and Phytobiotics

Now we move from probiotics (the bacteria) and prebiotics (their food and fuel) to some newer ideas about gut health: postbiotics (the compounds our bacteria produce, such as short-chain fatty acids) and phytobiotics (plant extracts such as flavonoids that can help protect "good" bacteria and nutrients such as zinc carnosine that can improve gut integrity and help establish a healthy gut environment to grow a robust, diverse, and resilient microbiome). It is through these phyto- and postbiotics that the aforementioned Mediterranean diet pattern of eating (lots of brightly colored high-fiber fruits and vegetables balanced with moderate amounts of healthy proteins and fats) is thought to be exerting some of its most important health benefits—by feeding our microbiome (probiotics) the right fibers (prebiotics) and plant nutrients (phytobiotics) to optimize metabolic production of healthy signaling molecules (postbiotics). It all sounds very logical (now), but none of this was very well known until just a few years ago, and every day we are learning more and more about the entire process and how to optimize it all.

At this point, our list of postbiotics is fairly short, including primarily vitamins (notably all the B-complexes and vitamin K) and short-chain fatty acids (SCFAs) such as acetate, propionate, and especially butyrate that exert positive benefits on the intestinal mucosa and gut lining. Butyrate is a primary energy source for colonocytes (intestinal cells) and also maintains intestinal homeostasis through anti-inflammatory actions. At the cellular level, SCFAs can have wide-ranging effects, including anti-cancer and antidiabetic effects as well as general improvement of immune vigilance. Greater exposure to SCFAs, particularly butyrate, has been associated with lower rates of gut-brain axis dysfunction such as IBS, so it makes sense to both make more butyrate (by supplying our microbiome with prebiotic fibers) and take more butyrate (as a daily supplement such as complexes of calcium butyrate and magnesium butyrate).

Phytobiotics can help to optimize mental focus (directly in the brain as well as indirectly via the gut), balance normal immune/inflammatory function, and support viability of healthy gut bacteria.

Apple cultivation originated in central Asia thousands of years ago. While most of the apples we eat in America come from the states of Washington or New York, some of the most polyphenol-rich apples are still grown in the region of the world known as the "stans" (Kazakhstan, Kyrgyzstan, Tajikistan, Turkmenistan, and Uzbekistan) between the Caspian Sea to the east and Mongolia to the west. Apples are the most popular fruit in America, and while they can provide a rich source of quercetin (a polyphenol that has health benefits across the entire gut-heart-brain axis), the polyphenols extracted from wild green unripe apple fruits provide an optimized profile of procyanidins that can influence and modulate gut microbiota with potent prebiotic effects.

Grape seed polyphenols contain flavonoids, which are considered to have numerous biological properties, including but not limited to antioxidant, anti-inflammatory, anticancer, antimicrobial, antiviral, cardioprotective, neuroprotective, and hepatoprotective (liver) activities. Grape seed is particularly high in a class of polyphenols known as proanthocyanidins (PACs).

Pine bark polyphenols are produced from *Pinus radiata* bark from trees grown in the pristine, unpolluted environment of New Zealand's sustainable forest plantations. They are extremely high in oligomeric proanthocyanidins (OPCs) with antibacterial, antiviral, anticarcinogenic, antiaging, anti-inflammatory, and anti-allergic properties.

Benefits across these three different types of polyphenols include antioxidant/anti-inflammatory protection of delicate neurons (first brain); reshaping the gut microbiome, with particular improvement in *Akkermansia* species associated with a healthy gut lining (second brain); improved physical energy and heart function (third brain); and regulation of immune and nervous system function (axis).

Zinc/carnosine complex is a complex of the essential mineral zinc and the amino acid L-carnosine that helps to relieve occasional gastric discomfort. When zinc is complexed to L-carnosine, it dissociates in the stomach at a slow, controlled rate. This prolonged presence in the stomach allows it to maintain its gastric healing effect over a longer period of time. Zinc/carnosine may also help maintain the bacterial balance throughout the upper/middle/lower gastrointestinal tract with a "displacement" effect on certain strains of harmful bacteria. By supporting the bacterial balance in the stomach, it can also help maintain healthy mucosal tissues that may soothe irritated gastric linings in the middle (small intestine) and lower (large intestine) gastrointestinal tract to support overall microbiome balance.

Artichoke leaf and ginger root can be used separately and in combination with proven benefits in managing digestive discomforts and enhancing gastric motility. Artichoke leaves are proven to reduce stomach swelling and bloating, in addition to its action as an antidyspeptic (reducing indigestion and digestive upset). Ginger is proven to increase gastric emptying and combat nausea. The combination of ginger and artichoke has been shown in clinical studies to promote overall digestive function and help regulate gastrointestinal motility to reduce gas and bloating.

Glutamine is the most abundant amino acid in the bloodstream and is especially helpful in maintaining tight junctions to fight leaky gut. It serves as a primary energy source for enterocytes (intestinal cells) to rebuild and repair as well as an essential neurotransmitter in the brain that helps with memory, focus, and concentration. Optimal glutamine levels help to optimize communication within and between all parts of the entire gut-heart-brain axis by balancing levels and activity of signaling molecules (cytokines, neurotransmitters, and hormones) to optimize interactions among cells of the gut (enterocytes), immune system (macrophages), and brain (neurons).

Senna leaf has been used in India for thousands of years as a laxative, resulting in intestinal contractions that can enhance elimination. Because of this ability, senna leaf is helpful in relieving constipation, often leading to bowel movements within six to twelve hours after ingestion. In traditional Chinese medicine, senna leaf "removes heat" from the colon, helping get rid of waste, and is often included in a variety of "detox" supplements.

Aloe vera leaf grows wild in tropical climates around the world. It increases intestinal water content, stimulates mucus secretion, and increases intestinal peristalsis—all of which combine to deliver the general "soothing" benefits attributed to aloe.

Traditionally, Native Americans used yellow dock root to help allevi-ate constipation and "cleanse" the blood. Used as a general "detoxifier," especially for the liver, yellow dock helps to stimulate bile production, which helps digestion, particularly of fats. Yellow dock root can stimulate bowel movements but is generally used more to help alleviate gastric reflux, excess stomach acid, heartburn, and indigestion. It stimulates digestive function by helping to increase digestive enzymes in both the stomach and small intestines.

Burdock root has been an important botanical in Western folk herb-alism and traditional Chinese medicine for thousands of years, primarily valued for its "cleansing" (liver support) and digestive properties. High concentration of fibers in burdock helps to stimulate the digestive system and moves food smoothly through the bowels, relieving constipation and preventing bloating, cramping, and ulcers. Inulin, a particular type of pre-biotic fiber found in burdock, is able to reduce inflammation in the gut and support growth of healthy bacteria.

Cayenne fruit is a well-known circulatory stimulant and digestive aid across many systems of traditional medicine. It increases the pulse of our lymphatic and digestive rhythms. Cayenne pepper is helpful for relieving intestinal gas and especially aids in protein digestion, possibly due to improvements in hydrochloric acid production.

Supplements to Support the Head Brain

When most people think about supplements to improve brain function, they tend to think of stimulants such as caffeine to help "amp up" brain function. This can certainly be an effective approach, but only up to a point. Supplements intended to improve cognitive function, memory, focus, and other aspects of brain performance are sometimes referred to as "nootropics"—pronounced "noah-tropic" and derived from the ancient Greek words *noos* (mind) and *trope* (a turning) to suggest a "turning of the mind" toward higher mental performance. The most common noo-tropics, of course, are the multitude of energy drinks comprising various combinations of caffeine, sugar, vitamins, amino acids, and artificial flavors. Let me be clear about what I think of energy drinks—they are for idiots.

Energy Drinks Are for Morons

I know, I should not be so flippant, but the billions of dollars people spend every year on energy drinks are largely wasted, because the products are so mismatched for the job they are intended to do as to be comparable to using a screwdriver to pound a nail. You could get the job done that way, but it is not very effective and there are much better ways. Using an energy drink to improve your brain function is a lot like using an antidepressant drug to improve your mood—neither works very well because you are using a tool that was intended for a different job. The antidepressant does not help you "feel better"; it helps you "feel less bad" (because it blocks feelings of sadness, which is completely different from boosting happiness). Likewise, the caffeine/sugar concoction in the energy drink does not help your brain work better or increase your mental energy; it only helps you "feel less fatigued" (because the caffeine and sugar blend blocks sensations of fatigue). These nuances might sound like wordplay, but they are actually extremely important distinctions related to how different compounds work across our gut-heart-brain axis and ultimately how they help us reach our peak mental fitness.

The nootropic category is popular and growing rapidly to encompass not just caffeine but a variety of supplements and drugs such as nicotine, methylphenidate (Ritalin for ADHD), and modafinil (Provigil for narcolepsy) that are sometimes referred to as "smart drugs" and are increasingly used by harried students, stressed workers, and tired moms. All of these stimulant drugs carry a significant risk of dependence, addiction, and serious adverse side effects.

The use of cholinergics is one of the most popular approaches to boosting brain function, with the intent of boosting production of acetylcholine (the brain's primary executive neurotransmitter needed for memory, focus, creativity, and virtually every aspect of mental performance). Most of these supplements are different analogues of choline (an essential nutrient similar to B-complex vitamins needed as a building block for acetylcholine production). Supplements of choline or its more stable form, choline bitartrate, can bolster dietary intake of choline, but it does not seem to noticeably boost mental performance the way choline compounds have been shown to do. For example, both citicoline (cytidine + choline) and alpha-glycerylphosphorylcholine (alpha-GPC) have been shown in clinical trials to improve focus, memory, and a wide range of "executive functions" (broadly defined as "managing oneself and one's resources in order to achieve a goal").

A wide array of herbal extracts fall into the nootropic category because they can help improve focus (ginkgo and bacopa) and reduce stress (ginseng and sage). Consider for a moment the different polyphenols (from apples, grape seeds, and pine bark) outlined earlier to support our gut brain; these are routinely used around the world to enhance mental focus (as natural ADHD treatments in kids) and alleviate dementia-related memory problems (in older adults), so these supplements could be considered as effective for "head brain" support as much as they are considered "gut brain" support. This is a scenario that we will come back to again and again, where one supplement might have myriad benefits across numerous parts of the gut-heart-brain axis, making it difficult to confine certain supplements to only one "box."

Coffee and Tea

Polyphenols are a broad category of thousands of related compounds naturally found in plant foods, such as fruits, vegetables, herbs, spices, dark chocolate, and wine. But by far the richest concentration of polyphenols in our diet is a drink that most of us consume every day—coffee and tea.

Coffee and tea are the most popular drinks around the globe (number three and number two in total consumption after water). Despite both of them delivering profound health benefits—including anticancer, antidiabetic, and anti-Alzheimer's effects—people tend to think of them primarily for their mental and physical "performance" benefits (energy, focus, alertness). Coffee in particular is sometimes thought of as unhealthy (even though it is packed with polyphenols that support our entire gut-heart-brain axis) because it is very easy to overdo our caffeine intake, which can lead to irritability, nervousness, anxiety, tension, heart palpitations, and insomnia. Of course, it's not that coffee is "bad" (quite the opposite actually—it is one of the healthiest drinks on the planet) but rather that we need to judiciously monitor our caffeine intake so that we get enough to induce the mental/physical benefits (around 200 mg/day) but not so much that it causes problems with tension and anxiety (around 400 mg/day).

A lot of people who have the mistaken notion that coffee is unhealthy will try to switch over to drinking tea for its perceived healthy aura. In general, tea has about half the caffeine content of coffee (but a lot of that depends on the variety of coffee or tea and how each is brewed), so a very rough rule of thumb is that a cup of tea provides about 50 mg of caffeine while a cup of coffee provides about 100 mg (although a typical Starbucks Grande might contain 200 to 250 mg in a single cup). Green tea (*Camellia sinensis*) in particular has been used medicinally for centuries in India and China. The active constituents in green tea are a family of polyphenols (catechins) with antioxidant activity about twenty-five to one hundred times more potent than vitamins C and E. A cup of green tea may provide 10 to 40 mg of polyphenols and has antioxidant activity greater than a serving of broccoli, spinach, carrots, or strawberries. Because the catechins found in green tea possess potent antioxidant and anti-inflammatory activity, population studies have shown a significantly lower risk for inflammatory conditions, especially dementia and Alzheimer's, in people who drink several cups of tea (or coffee) daily.

Theanine

One of the advantages that tea holds over coffee is that tea leaves also contain theanine, which is an amino acid with profound benefits for reducing stress and promoting focus—what I refer to as "relaxed alertness" (also known as being "in the zone"). Theanine offers quite different benefits from those imparted by the polyphenol and catechin antioxidants for which green tea is typically consumed. In fact, through the natural production of polyphenols, the tea plant converts theanine into catechins. This means tea leaves harvested during one part of the growing season may be high in catechins (good for anti-inflammatory and antidementia benefits), while leaves harvested during another time of year may be higher in theanine (good for anti-stress and mental focus effects). Theanine is unique in that it acts as a nonsedating relaxant to help increase the brain's production of alpha waves. This makes theanine extremely effective for combating tension, stress, and anxiety, without inducing drowsiness. Clinical studies show that theanine is effective in dosages ranging from 50 to 200 mg per day. A typical cup of green tea is expected to contain approximately 50 mg of theanine (balanced with 50 mg of caffeine for the ultimate in focused alertness without tension and jitters). In addition to being considered a relaxing substance (in adults), theanine has also been shown to provide benefits for improving learning performance (in mice) and promoting concentration (in students). No adverse side effects are associated with theanine consumption, making it one of the leading natural choices for promoting relaxation without the sedating effects of depressant drugs and herbs. When considering the potential benefits of theanine as an anti-stress or biochemical-balance supplement, it is important to distinguish its nonsedating relaxation benefits from the tranquilizing effects of other "relaxing" supplements, such as valerian and kava, which are actually mild central nervous system depressants (which might be useful for inducing sleep but not appropriate for daytime usage).

One of the most distinctive aspects of theanine activity is its ability to increase the brain's output of alpha waves. Alpha waves are one of the four basic brain wave patterns (delta, theta, alpha, and beta) that can be monitored using an electroencephalogram (EEG). Each wave pattern is associated with a particular oscillating electrical voltage in the brain, and the different brain wave patterns are associated with different mental states and states of consciousness. Alpha waves, which indicate what we call "relaxed alertness," are nonexistent during deep sleep as well as during states of very high arousal, such as fear or anger. In other words, alpha waves are associated with your highest levels of mental fitness and physical performance; therefore, you want to maximize the amount of time during your waking hours that your brain spends in an alpha state. By increasing the brain's output of alpha waves, theanine can help us "rebalance" our brain wave patterns as well as help us control anxiety, increase focus and concentration, promote creativity, and improve overall mental fitness and physical performance. Research studies have clearly shown that people who produce more alpha brain waves also have less anxiety, that highly creative people generate more alpha waves when faced with a problem to solve, and that elite athletes tend to produce a burst of alpha waves on the left sides of their brains during their best performances.

Matcha Tea

Matcha tea (whole-leaf green tea that has been dried and powdered) is gaining popularity throughout the world in recent years and is frequently referred to as a mood-and-brain food. Previous research has demonstrated that three constituents present in matcha tea—theanine, epigallocatechin gallate (EGCG), and caffeine—affect mood and cognitive performance. Matcha tea can induce significant benefits on speed of attention and overall memory because it provides a higher intake of phytochemicals compared to regular brewed green tea. For example, studies show quite clearly that the individual components of green tea have unique benefits—catechins such as EGCG have anti-inflammatory benefits, caffeine has arousal benefits, and theanine has relaxation benefits—but that the combination of phytochemicals (as found in matcha) has significantly superior mental fitness benefits in "attention switching" tasks that tend to dominate our day (answering emails, attending meetings, caring for children, solving problems, writing, reading, speaking, and the like).

Two additional, and extremely important, benefits shared by polyphenols and theanine are that they can both increase levels of BDNF in the hippocampus (memory center) of the brain and reduce cortisol (stress hormone) exposure—both of which are highly related to improved mental fitness and optimal brain performance (more on BDNF to follow).

Branched-Chain Amino Acids (BCAAs)

Continuing the theme of "brain foods" such as coffee and tea—and amino acids such as theanine—let us now consider the group of three essential amino acids referred to as the "branched-chain amino acids" (BCAAs): valine, leucine, and isoleucine. BCAAs are found in high levels in protein-containing foods such as beef, chicken, turkey, eggs, and milk, but they can also be found in plant-derived proteins such as rice, hemp, peas, and chickpeas (my favorite source). Supplemental levels of BCAAs have been shown to increase endurance, reduce fatigue, improve mental performance, increase energy levels, prevent immune system suppression, and counteract the catabolism (breakdown) of muscles and gut linings following intense exercise. In numerous studies of athletes, BCAAs have been shown to maintain blood levels of glutamine, an amino acid used as fuel by immune system cells and gut-lining cells (enterocytes). During intense exercise and stress, glutamine levels typically fall dramatically, removing the primary fuel source for immune/intestinal cells and leading to a general suppression of immune system activity, an increased risk of infections, and an increase in gut-related problems such as leaky gut. By supplementing with glutamine, BCAAs, or both, a person can not only avoid these problems but also find a ready source of fuel that directly improves metabolism across the entire gut-heart-brain axis for superior mental fitness. In related studies, BCAA supplements have also been shown to help counteract the rise in cortisol and the drop in testosterone that is often seen during a variety of high-stress situations, such as athletes undergoing stressful training, workers under deadlines, and caregivers experiencing sleep deprivation.

Ashwagandha

Ashwagandha (*Withania somnifera*) is an herb from India that is some-times called "Indian ginseng"—not because it is part of the ginseng family but to suggest energy-promoting and anti-stress benefits that are similar to the ones attributed to the more well-known Asian and Siberian ginsengs. Traditional use of ashwagandha in Indian (Ayurvedic) medicine is to "balance life forces" during stress and aging, similar to the use of cordyceps in restoring "qi" (pronounced "chee") in traditional Chinese medicine and the modern use of many of these "adaptogenic" supplements for restoring vigor in modern nutritional psychology. The active ingredients in ashwagandha (withanolides) are thought to contribute to its calming effects during periods of stress and may account for the use of ashwagandha as a general tonic during stressful situations (where it is calming) and as a treatment for insomnia (where it promotes relaxation).

Magnolia Bark

Magnolia bark (*Magnolia officinalis*) is a traditional Chinese medicine used since CE 100 for treating "stagnation of qi," what we view in Western medicine as low vigor or burnout. Magnolia bark extracts are rich in two biphenyl compounds, magnolol and honokiol, both of which are thought to contribute to the primary anti-stress and cortisol-lowering effects of the plant. Researchers in Japan and America have shown both magnolol and honokiol to possess powerful "mental acuity" benefits via their actions in modulating the activity of various neurotransmitters and related enzymes in the brain (increased choline acetyltransferase activity, inhibition of acetylcholinesterase, and increased acetylcholine release), so magnolia bark certainly qualifies to be listed among the most effective of the nootropic-style supplements discussed earlier. Numerous animal studies have demonstrated that honokiol acts as a central nervous system depressant at high doses but as an anxiolytic (antianxiety and anti-stress) agent at lower doses. This means that a small dose of a magnolia bark extract standardized for honokiol content can help to "de-stress" a person, while a larger dose might have the effect of putting you to sleep. When compared to pharmaceutical agents such as Valium (diazepam), honokiol appears to be as effective in its antianxiety activity yet not nearly as powerful in its sedative ability. These results have been demonstrated in at least a half dozen animal studies and suggest that magnolia bark extracts standardized for honokiol content would be an appropriate approach for controlling the detrimental effects of everyday stressors, without the tranquilizing side effects of pharmaceutical agents.

Saffron

Spanish and Australian researchers have shown that saffron improves anxiety and depressive symptoms in teenagers and adults with mild to moderate symptoms of stress, anxiety, and depression. In other research, saffron extracts have been shown to be as effective as the drug methylphenidate (Ritalin) in treatment of kids (six to seventeen years old) with ADHD. This is important because as many as half of all children treated with ADHD stimulants cannot tolerate the side effects. Additionally, Iranian researchers have found saffron extracts to be as effective as fluoxetine (Prozac) in treating mild to moderate depression in adults. The main active compounds in saffron (lepticrosalides) have been associated with a wide range of improvements across many mental fitness–related behaviors, including normalizing neurotransmitter activity (serotonin, dopamine, norepinephrine/noradrenaline, GABA) and overall neuroprotection (reducing oxidative stress, inflammatory stress, and cortisol exposure).

While saffron might be the culinary spice with the highest degree of scientific evidence for specific mental fitness benefits, especially for treating depression and ADHD, sage is a close second (especially effective for anti-stress effects and mental focus improvements in dementia). Other spices can be generally supportive of overall brain function because of their potent antioxidant and anti-inflammatory effects, such as rosemary (memory), clove (anxiety), oregano (fatigue), and holy basil (stress).

Guayusa Leaf

Guayusa (pronounced "gwhy-you-sa") is an Amazonian evergreen tree native to South America and particularly in the upper Amazonian region of Ecuador and Peru. The leaves contain a small amount of naturally occurring caffeine that is balanced with diverse polyphenols and carotenoids as well as more than a dozen amino acids. This unique combination of nutrients delivers a clean, focused energy that indigenous users say helps them "connect with the universe"—what modern nutrition psychologists might refer to as "mental awareness." Guayusa is traditionally referred to as the "night watchman" by native hunters, because consuming it before night hunts helps them stay awake, alert, and aware of their surroundings.

Pomegranate Extract

Pomegranate extract is among the "smartest fruits" that you could possibly add to your diet, because it optimizes function across all parts of the gut-heart-brain axis. In particular, pomegranate extracts have been shown to enhance overall brain activation, promote higher brain blood flow, and stimulate bilateral activation of the hippocampus (area of the brain involved in memory). Studies are underway to explore a range of pomegranate compounds, including one called punicalagin, that have shown early evidence for improving memory and slowing the progression of Alzheimer's and Parkinson's disease. Interestingly, it seems that the synergistic action of the broad range of pomegranate constituents appears to be superior to that of single constituents, especially for stimulation of neuron growth and overall brain plasticity.

Pine Bark Extract

Pine bark extract is a polyphenol-rich ingredient mentioned earlier for support of our gut brain, but I want to come back to it again here because of its profound benefits for our head brain. Pine bark is particularly high in a class of polyphenols known as oligomeric proanthocyanidins (OPCs), which have been shown to be effective in treating both ADHD (getting the brain to work better in terms of focused concentration) and restoring cognitive function after traumatic brain injuries, such as concussions, by accelerating the repair of damaged neurons and restoring connections across the brain's neural network. In New Zealand, pine bark is very often used as first-line treatment for ADHD in children and adults, and clinical studies have shown improvements in working memory, cognitive function, and overall mental performance. Pine bark can be sourced from different species of pine trees in North and Central America, Europe, Asia, and New Zealand. I prefer to use varieties of the *Pinus radiata* species that flourishes in certain parts of Central America and New Zealand because the starting material is of the highest purity and the extraction methods involve only hot water to concentrate the OPCs. In certain extracts from Europe, there is detectable solvent residue from the extraction process, and many Chinese extracts suffer from the pine bark raw material being contaminated with heavy metals, environmental toxins, and beetle infestations—none of which you want to include in a supplement intended for brain protection and mental fitness improvement.

Rafuma

Rafuma (*Apocynum venetum*) is a small shrub, the leaves of which make a tea that is particularly popular in China and has been used in traditional Chinese medicine for thousands of years (as the medicine "Luo Bu Ma Ye"). Commonly called sword-leaf dogbane, rafuma is used to "soothe the nerves, calm the liver, and dissipate heat" (which are all slightly different explanations in TCM for a reduction in depression and inflammation with improvements in mood). The first recorded use was in the Ming Dynasty in the ancient fifteenth-century Chinese herbal book *Jiuhuang Bencao*. The *Compendium of Materia Medica*, which also was written in the fifteenth century, states that the herb eliminates "dampness" (water retention) through diuresis. In modern times, rafuma is also known as luobuma in China, and the Chinese Pharmacopoeia recommends it for a wide range of what we in Western society would view as anti-stress and mood-elevating effects. It is also listed in ancient texts for treating neurasthenia (anxiety and depression), palpitation, insomnia, and hypertension and even for detoxifying nicotine, with potential benefits for helping people quit smoking and reduce use of other addictive substances. Its mechanism of action appears to be via GABA and serotonin pathways with primary bioactive compounds including quercetin and hyperoside.

Kanna

Kanna (*Sceletium tortuosum*) is one of my absolute favorite natural ingredients for reducing stress, for boosting mood, and especially for enhancing stress resilience. Kanna is a small cactus-like succulent that is traditionally used by the San and Khoi peoples of Southern Africa as an analgesic (pain reliever), sedative, tonic (energy/stamina), and mood elevator. The traditionally prepared dried plant material is chewed, smoked, or powdered and inhaled as a snuff. It is also used as a tea or tincture. It was typically used in cognitively stressing situations, such as hunting, during which its "adaptogenic" (stress-balancing) properties are readily apparent. Lower daily doses are known to have a subtle effect, providing a sense of serenity and at the same time an elevated sense of alertness and awareness, while larger doses lead to a transient euphoria. Used as a daily stress resilience supplement, kanna delivers a wide range of positive health benefits, including elevated mood and mental clarity, improved focus and memory, increased energy and motivation, lower stress hormone levels, and decreased everyday anxiety. Kanna contains a family of alkaloids (mesembrine, mesembrenone, mesembrenol, and mesembranol) confirmed to provide the multifactorial mechanisms responsible for the dramatic mood-elevating and anti-stress benefits. Kanna is known to influence the amygdala of the brain (a brain region central in emotional processing and fear/stress responses) and is known to have modulatory effects on serotonin, GABA, dopamine, acetylcholine, and norepinephrine pathways. This places kanna in a very unique position among natural ingredients for supporting mental fitness because it works across the entire mental fitness continuum from depression and anxiety (helping you feel normal again) to stress and fatigue (helping you feel as good as you ever have) to resilience and optimization (helping you "level up" to heights of mental fitness and physical performance that previously seemed out of reach).

Corn Grass

Corn grass (*Zea mays*) is just what it sounds like—the "grass" that develops into a corn plant. If you have ever seen the wheatgrass on display at your local smoothie shop, then you have seen a related "monocot grass" that contains a specialized phytonutrient (methoxybenzoxazolinone, or MBOA), which acts as a positive regulator of the serotonin/melatonin system to enhance daytime serotonin levels (for mood improvement) and nighttime melatonin synthesis (for improved sleep quality). Corn grass has been clinically shown to address both mental and mood imbalances and to provide sleep-improvement benefits that are superior to melatonin-based sleep aids. I am not a big fan of using synthetic melatonin supplements to induce sleep (especially for kids and teens), because melatonin works for only about half of people who try it, and those it does work for often wake up with the common "melatonin hangover" because their body has not fully metabolized their melatonin dose overnight, so they spend the first half of the day in a groggy melatonin-induced brain fog (not exactly what they were hoping to get from a sleep aid). In addition, regular or frequent use of melatonin supplements can induce a dependence where your body stops producing this hormone on its own and must rely on nightly supplements to sleep at all. Corn grass helps your body and brain naturally produce its own melatonin on demand, in the right amounts at the right time. Doing so has been shown to improve the amount of time spent in REM sleep (where the brain repairs) and deep sleep (where the body recovers) by as much as 40 percent. Combining corn grass with a small amount of Griffonia seed is a way to naturally supply the amino acid 5-hydroxytryptophan (5-HTP) that is used as a building block for the production of serotonin and melatonin—and nutrient cofactors vitamin B6, C, zinc, and magnesium to optimize serotonin/melatonin metabolism. Griffonia seeds are native to the Western and Central regions of Africa, where they are used medicinally to treat a wide range of stress-induced problems. I often recommend the combination of corn grass and Griffonia seed for not just enhancing sleep quality but also for addressing stress-related imbalances, including issues like insomnia, depression, anxiety, sugar cravings, and pain (including fibromyalgia and migraine).

Japanese Asparagus

Japanese asparagus extract is a rich source of unique phytonutrients with the special ability to help the body create Hsp70 (heat shock protein 70), which is a cellular protein that helps protect cells (especially delicate neurons) from stressors, repairs damaged cells, and balances inflammatory cytokine responses. This biochemical reaction improves cognitive performance, reduces fatigue, and improves stress response. Unfortunately, our heat shock protein response to stressors of all kinds decreases with age but is also thought to be one of the most modifiable "antiaging" pathways that we can actively manage to help maintain mental fitness and physical health as we age. Clinical research has shown that Japanese asparagus extract significantly increases the expression of Hsp70 and is effective in modifying stress responses, improving sleep quality, and improving HRV (so here is another example of a "brain" supplement that also has important benefits for another part of the gut-heart-brain axis).

Supplements to Support the Heart Brain

When we think of "heart health" supplements, we tend to gravitate toward those that lower cholesterol such as oat bran and psyllium fiber or those that might improve the contractile function of the heart such as coenzyme Q10, carnitine, and ribose. These are all logical choices, but when we are focusing specifically on the heart as our "third brain" and as a factor in our mental fitness, we want to instead think about how we can improve the electromagnetic signals that the heart brain sends to our head brain and to the rest of our body. We also want to think about supplements that can help to control inflammation, because inflammatory cytokines are one of the predominant signaling pathways from the heart to the brain and are directly related to heart function. As such, I will cover it here even though we could also think of the inflammatory cascade as a communication system within the "axis" portion of the gut-heart-brain axis.

Essential Fatty Acids

The term *essential fatty acids* refers to two fatty acids—linoleic acid and alpha-linolenic acid—that the body cannot synthesize and thus must be consumed in the diet. (Vitamins and minerals are also termed "essential," because the body cannot make them and therefore must consume them.) These essential fatty acids are needed for the production of compounds known as cytokines, which help regulate inflammation, blood clotting, blood pressure, heart rate, immune response, and a wide variety of other biological processes, including getting signals across the blood-brain barrier.

Linoleic acid is considered an omega-6 (n-6) fatty acid. It is found in vegetable and nut oils such as sunflower, safflower, corn, soy, and peanut oil. Most Americans get adequate levels of these omega-6 oils in their diets due to a high consumption of vegetable oil–based margarine, salad dressings, and processed convenience foods. Alpha-linolenic acid is classified as an omega-3 (n-3) fatty acid. Good dietary sources are flax-seed oil (51 percent alpha-linolenic acid), soy oil (7 percent), walnuts (7 percent), and canola oil (9 percent) as well as margarine derived from canola oil. For example, a tablespoon of canola oil or canola oil margarine provides about 1 gram of alpha-linolenic acid.

If you think back to the type of diet humans evolved to eat, it provided a much more balanced mix of n-3 and n-6 fatty acids. Over the last century, modern diets have come to rely heavily on fats derived from vegetable oils (n-6), bringing the ratio of n-6 to n-3 fatty acids from our ancestors' ratio of 1:1 to the modern-day range of 20:1 or 30:1! This highly unbalanced intake of high n-6 fatty acids and low n-3 fatty acids sets the stage for increases in various inflammatory processes. Fatty acids of the n-3 variety have opposing biological effects to the n-6 fatty acids, meaning that a higher intake of n-3 oils can deliver anti-inflammatory, antithrombotic, and vasodilatory effects that can lead to benefits in terms of heart disease, hypertension, diabetes, and a wide variety of inflammatory conditions, such as fibromyalgia, rheumatoid arthritis, ulcerative colitis, and depression.

In the body, linoleic acid (n-6) is metabolized into arachidonic acid, a precursor to specific "bad" cytokines that can promote vasoconstriction, elevated blood pressure, and painful inflammation, while the n-3 fatty acids eicosapentaenoic acid (EPA) and docosahexaenoic acid (DHA) serve as the precursors to anti-inflammatory prostaglandins, which can counteract the inflammation caused by n-6 fatty acids. Recent studies have shown that consumption of alpha-linolenic acid and other n-3 fatty acids offers wide-ranging anti-inflammatory benefits. This effect is thought to be mediated through the synthesis of EPA and DHA. Fish oils contain large amounts of EPA and DHA, and the majority of studies in this area have used various concentrations of fish oil supplements to demonstrate the health benefits of these essential fatty acids. Some evidence suggests that omega-3 fatty acids from fish oil and flaxseed can reduce perception of stress, with a ratio of 5:1 EPA to DHA being shown to be particularly effective for enhancing mental fitness parameters such as depression and anxiety.

Fish Oil

The best dietary sources of omega-3 fatty acids are fish, such as trout, tuna, salmon, mackerel, herring, and sardines, which all contain 1 to 2 grams of n-3 oils per three- to four-ounce serving. A minimum of 4 to 5 grams of linoleic acid (but no more than 6 to 7 grams) and 2 to 3 grams of alpha-linolenic acid are recommended per day. Supplements of linoleic acid (n-6) are typically not needed, whereas alpha-linolenic acid (n-3) supplements (4 to 10 g per day) or concentrated EPA/DHA supplements (400 to 1,000 mg per day) are recommended to balance normal inflammatory processes. In addition to fish oils, other plant-derived oils can be rich sources of essential fatty acids, including flaxseed, borage seed, and evening primrose.

Evening Primrose Oil

Evening primrose oil (EPO) is most commonly used for relieving inflammatory conditions associated with "women's health," such as premenstrual syndrome (PMS), fibrocystic breasts, and menopausal symptoms, such as hot flashes. Each of these conditions is related on a biochemical level to an excessive inflammatory response. EPO contains a unique form of linoleic acid, gamma linoleic acid (GLA), that is important for controlling inflammation. The body synthesizes GLA from linoleic acid, which comprises 8 to 14 percent of the oil in EPO supplements. GLA is a precursor of prostaglandin E1 (PGE1), a deficiency of which has been documented in some women with PMS and cyclical breast pain. Because decreased levels of PGE1 can increase the pain-inducing effect of the hormone prolactin on breast tissue, it is thought that they may be a primary cause of many of the symptoms associated with PMS.

Borage Seeds

Borage seeds are also a rich source of GLA (20 to 30 percent of total oil content), which has medicinal properties that have been demonstrated in such areas as anti-inflammatory activity, immune system modulation, management of atopic eczema (excessive proliferation of the skin cells), and other skin maladies. Studies have shown that individuals with active rheumatoid arthritis (an inflammatory condition) experienced an improvement in their symptoms when they were given a borage oil supplement daily for six months.

Flaxseed Oil

Flaxseed oil is just what it sounds like—oil from the seed of the flax plant. Flaxseed is typically used as a source of the essential fatty acids alpha-linolenic acid (ALA) and linoleic acid (LA). Flaxseed oil is about 57 percent ALA (an omega-3) and about 17 percent LA (an omega-6). ALA can be converted into EPA and DHA, fatty acids that are precursors to anti-inflammatory prostaglandins. Regular flaxseed consumption has been associated with improvements in the ratio of omega-3 to omega-6 fatty acids in the blood, a situation that may offer protection and relief from inflammatory conditions. A number of animal and human studies on flaxseed oil have shown a clear and consistent reduction in pro-inflammatory markers (tumor necrosis factor and interleukins).

Ginger

Ginger (*Zingiber officinale*) has been used throughout history as an aid for many gastrointestinal disturbances as well as for relief of inflamed joints and as a general "heart tonic" to reduce fatigue. The most active chemical compounds in ginger are known as the gingerols, which are also the most aromatic compounds in this root and are thought to be the reason that ginger can inhibit substances that cause the pain and inflammation associated with osteoarthritis. Ginger supplementation is known to reduce production of the inflammatory thromboxane compounds associated with excess inflammation and pain. In studies of patients with osteoarthritis and rheumatoid arthritis, significant pain relief was noted in more than half (55 percent) of the osteoarthritis patients and nearly three-quarters (74 percent) of the rheumatoid arthritis patients when supplemented with ginger.

Turmeric

Turmeric is known by the Latin plant name *Curcuma longa* (where the name for the turmeric-derived spice "curcumin" comes from) and is a member of the ginger family (Zingiberaceae). As a traditional medicine, turmeric is used as an anti-inflammatory, antioxidant, and analgesic (pain reliever). Currently, research is continuing to investigate turmeric's anti-inflammatory effects and its potential as a potent anticancer agent (which makes sense if cancer is viewed as a disease of both too much inflammation and too little immune vigilance). The primary active compounds in turmeric are the flavonoid curcumin and related "curcuminoid" compounds that deliver potent antioxidant, anti-inflammatory, and chemopreventive (anticancer) effects. As such, turmeric-containing supplements would logically be expected to have a beneficial effect in such areas as arthritis, cancer, and heart disease. In a wide range of animal studies, turmeric extracts have been shown to significantly alleviate the physical pain of arthritis as well as the mental pain of depression.

Boswellia

The boswellia plant (*Boswellia serrata*), also known as frankincense, produces a sap that has been used in traditional Indian medicine as a treatment for arthritis, inflammatory conditions, and mood disorders. The primary compounds thought to be responsible for the anti-inflammatory activity of boswellia are known as boswellic acids. These compounds are known to interfere with enzymes that contribute to inflammation and pain. Boswellia sap/resin has a long history of safe and effective use as a mild anti-inflammatory to reduce pain and stiffness and promote increased mobility (without many of the associated gastrointestinal side effects commonly reported for synthetic anti-inflammatory medications). A number of studies have shown that boswellic acids may possess anti-inflammatory activity at least as potent as common over-the-counter medications such as ibuprofen and aspirin.

Nutmeg

The nutmeg (*Myristica fragrans*) that you might know as a "holiday spice" is derived from seeds from evergreen trees native to the rainforest of Indonesia, known as the "Spice Islands." The aromatic oil from the seeds is a key principle active in herbal medicine for treating a wide range of gut-heart-brain axis dysfunctions, including infections, depression, low sex drive, and digestive complaints such as gas and constipation.

Astragalus

Also known as "Huang Qi" in traditional Chinese medicine, astragalus is an amazing root that is considered to be a sweet tonic herb that is "slightly warming," to describe its main benefits as a mildly stimulating energizer and immune-enhancing adaptogen. It has a high content of triterpenoid saponin glycosides known as astragalosides, in addition to polysaccharide glucans and heteroglycans, that broadly contribute to the reputation of astragalus as a "qi tonic" (qi = life force) that encourages a general state of tranquility and positive mood by improving both mental and physical stress resilience.

Poria Cocos

A medicinal mushroom, also called "Fu Ling" in traditional Chinese medicine, poria is known as the "fungus of immortality." The major constituent of poria is a unique polysaccharide in the form of beta-glucan, which we will cover in more detail in the next section about supplements to support the axis and particularly the immune system. Variable biological functions have been reported for poria cocos polysaccharides, such as antioxidant, antihyperglycemic, soothing stomach pain, anti-inflammation, anticancer, and immunological modulation. Practitioners of traditional Chinese medicine believe in the concept of *shen*—which translates roughly to "mind" or "spirit"—and believe that poria is able to target disturbances within a person's shen to relieve stress and induce a calming effect on the mind and body of those who use it.

Bromelain and Papain

The word *proteolytic* is a catchall term referring to enzymes that digest protein. In the body, proteolytic enzymes—such as bromelain (from pineapples) and papain (from papayas)—act as anti-inflammatory agents and pain relievers. They have been effective in accelerating recovery from exercise and injury in athletes as well as tissue repair in patients following surgery, including heart surgery. A number of clinical trials have shown proteolytic enzymes can help reduce inflammation, speed healing of bruises and other soft tissue injuries, and reduce overall recovery time following both physically and mentally stressful events.

Citrus Peel

The peels of a variety of citrus fruits, including oranges, tangerines, grapefruits, lemons, and limes (especially *Citrus sinensis* species) contain a unique class of flavonoids, known as polymethoxylated fla-vones (PMFs)—specifically tangeretin, sinensetin, and nobiletin. The PMFs represent a class of "superflavonoids" extracted from citrus peels that exhibit approximately threefold potency compared to other flavo-noids in terms of their anti-stress effects, both mentally and physically. PMFs are just what they sound like—flavonoid compounds with extra "methoxy" groups compared to "regular" flavones. Like all flavonoids, the PMFs deliver potent antioxidant and anti-inflammatory activity, but the PMF version is about three times more potent in its ability to reduce stress hormones and restore stress resilience. Our research group was the first in the world to use PMFs from citrus peel extract for restoring stress hormone balance while also promoting blood sugar control and weight loss. As part of several research trials, we provided supplements of PMFs (combined with eurycoma root extract, covered next) to a group of moderately stressed overweight subjects. The PMFs reduced cortisol levels by 20 percent, body weight by 5 percent, body fat by 6 percent, and waist circumference by 8 percent over a period of six weeks. A longer, twelve-week study showed even better results, with additional beneficial effects on reducing cholesterol (by 20 percent), boosting psychological vigor (by 25 percent), reducing fatigue (by 48 percent), and maintaining normal testosterone levels and resting metabolic rate at pre-weight loss levels (when they are expected to fall).

Eurycoma

Eurycoma longifolia, a Malaysian root often called "Malaysian ginseng" for its energy-boosting effects, affords a natural way to bring suboptimal testosterone levels back to within normal ranges. It is also probably the best first-line therapy (before trying synthetic options, such as DHEA supplements or topical/injected testosterone) for anybody suffering from chronic stress (which increases cortisol and decreases testosterone lev-els). In traditional Malaysian medicine, eurycoma is used as an antiaging remedy because of its positive effects on energy levels and mental out-look. Eurycoma contains a group of small peptides (short protein chains), referred to as "eurypeptides," that are known to have effects in improving energy status and sex drive. The "testosterone-boosting" effects of eurycoma appear not to have anything to do with stimulating testosterone synthesis but rather appear to increase the release rate of "free" testosterone from sex hormone–binding globulin. In this way, eurycoma is not so much a testosterone "booster" as a "maintainer" of normal testosterone levels (testosterone that your body has already produced and needs to release to become active). This means that eurycoma is particularly beneficial for individuals with suboptimal testosterone levels and low vigor, including those who are dieting for weight loss, middle-aged individuals (because testosterone drops after age thirty), stressed-out folks, sleep-deprived people, and serious athletes who may be at risk for overtraining. Suboptimal testosterone levels are also a primary risk factor for heart disease and heart attacks, so maintaining healthy testosterone levels is "heart healthy" in a variety of ways.

Ginseng

Ginseng is perhaps the best known of the adaptogens (herbs to help the body "adapt" to the biochemical imbalances caused by chronic stress). Several strains of ginseng are available—including *Panax ginseng* (true ginseng; also called Korean or Asian ginseng), American ginseng, and Siberian ginseng (not a true ginseng; see the next paragraph for more information)—and each type contains some of the same compounds but in slightly different proportions, thus providing slightly different effects in terms of anti-stress and mental fitness benefits. Numerous animal and human studies have shown that different types of ginseng can increase energy and endurance, improve mental function (learning and maze tests), and improve overall resistance to various stressors, including viruses and bacteria, extreme exercise, and sleep deprivation. Human studies have shown improved immune function and reduced incidence of colds and flu following a month of supplementation with *Panax ginseng*. In a handful of studies, ginseng supplementation has also provided benefits in mental functioning in volunteers exposed to stress, such as improvements in ability to form abstract thoughts, in reaction times, and in scores of tests of memory and concentration.

Siberian Ginseng

Also known as eleuthero (*Eleutherococcus senticosus*), Siberian ginseng is not truly ginseng, but it is a close-enough cousin to deliver some of the same energetic benefits. It is generally a less-expensive alternative to *Panax ginseng*, although it may have more of a stimulatory, energy-boosting effect rather than a balancing adaptogenic effect. This is not necessarily a bad thing if you just need a boost. Eleuthero is often promoted as an athletic performance enhancer because it can also promote recovery following intense exercise, perhaps due in part to an enhanced delivery of oxygen to recovering muscles (including the heart).

Cordyceps

Ounce for ounce more valuable than gold, cordyceps (*Cordyceps sinensis*) is a Chinese mushroom that has been used for centuries to reduce fatigue, increase stamina, improve heart and lung function (cardio-respiratory power), and restore qi (life force). Traditionally, it was harvested in the spring at elevations above fourteen thousand feet, which restricted its availability to the privileged (the emperor and his court). Several studies of cordyceps have shown improvements in heart and lung function, suggesting that athletes may benefit from an increased ability to take up and use oxygen. A handful of studies in stressed subjects have shown increases in libido (sex drive) and restoration of testosterone levels (from low to normal) following cordyceps supplementation. During stressful events, cortisol levels rise while testosterone levels drop, so using cordyceps as a way to normalize these suppressed testosterone levels can help modulate the cortisol-to-testosterone ratio within a lower (and healthier) range. At least two chemical constituents—cordycepin (3'-deoxyadenosine) and cordycepic acid (mannitol)—have been identified as the active compounds in improving energy and stamina. Animal studies have shown that feeding with cordyceps increases the level of adenosine triphosphate (ATP) in the liver by 45 to 55 percent, a beneficial effect for boosting energy state and potential for physical and mental performance. Furthermore, mice fed cordyceps and subjected to an extreme low-oxygen environment were able to utilize oxygen more efficiently (30 to 50 percent increase), better tolerate acidosis and hypoxia (lack of oxygen), and live two to three times longer than a control group. In a number of Chinese clinical studies, primarily in elderly patients with fatigue, cordyceps-treated patients reported significant improvements in their levels of fatigue, ability to tolerate cold temperatures, memory and cognitive capacity, and sex drive. Patients with respiratory diseases also reported feeling physically and mentally stronger. Recently, a small study presented at the American College of Sports Medicine's annual scientific conference showed that cordyceps significantly increased maximal oxygen uptake and anaerobic threshold, indicating enhanced heart-lung performance, which may lead to improved exercise capacity and resistance to fatigue.

Rhodiola

Rhodiola (*Rhodiola rosea*) is a species of plants from the arctic mountain regions of Tibet and Siberia. The root of the plant is also known as "arctic root" or "golden root." Rhodiola has been used for centuries to treat cold and flu-like symptoms, promote longevity, and increase the body's resistance to physical and mental stresses. It is typically considered to be an adaptogen (like ginseng) and is believed to invigorate the body and mind to increase resistance to a multitude of stresses. The key active constituents in rhodiola are believed to be rosavin, rosarin, rosin, and salidroside. In one clinical trial, rhodiola extract was effective in reducing or removing symptoms of depression in 65 percent of the patients studied (which is a significantly better rate of effectiveness compared to any of the prescription antidepressant drugs). In another study, 75 percent of men suffering from poor sexual performance reported improvements in sexual function following treatment with rhodiola extract for three months. In another study of physicians on nighttime hospital duty, rhodiola supplementation for two weeks resulted in a significant improvement in associative think-ing, short-term memory, concentration, and speed of audiovisual percep-tion. An additional study of students undergoing a stressful twenty-day period of exams showed daily rhodiola supplementation alleviated mental fatigue and improved well-being. Overall, rhodiola appears to be valuable as an adaptogen, specifically in increasing the body's ability to deal with a number of psychological and physiological stresses. Of particular value is the rhodiola's role in increasing the body's ability to take up and utilize oxygen—an effect similar to that of cordyceps—which may explain some of the non-stimulant "energizing" effects attributed to the plant. Rhodiola is often called the "poor man's cordyceps" because of ancient stories in which Chinese commoners and Tibetan Sherpas used rhodiola for energy because the plants grew wild throughout the countryside, while only the emperor, his immediate family, and his concubines were allowed access to the rare cordyceps mushroom.

Astaxanthin

Astaxanthin is a carotenoid derived from marine algae. It is the compound that makes shrimp look pink (and pink flamingos who eat the shrimp and algae). As a supplement, astaxanthin is known to promote brain health, provide cardiovascular support, decrease oxidative stress markers, and improve cognitive function. Recent clinical trials have shown that astax-anthin is particularly effective for supporting the heart-brain axis, where supplementation for one month resulted in improvements in heart rate at submaximal endurance intensities (suggesting a "physical" heart ben-efit) and improved mood state parameters (suggesting a "mental" brain benefit). While previous studies have shown astaxanthin supplementa-tion to improve parameters associated with heart health (antioxidant, fat oxidation, endurance, anti-fatigue) and brain health (neuroinflammation, cognition, antidepressant/anxiolytic), these most recent results suggest that natural astaxanthin supplementation supports the entire psycho-physiological "heart-brain axis" with simultaneous improvements in both physical and mental wellness.

Black Cumin Seed Oil

Also simply referred to as "black seed" (*Nigella sativa*), black cumin seed oil is known in traditional Middle Eastern medicine as the "immortality seed" that helps support blood sugar and cholesterol levels (both related to superior heart health) and enhances memory and cognitive health (obviously related to superior brain health). In addition, it favorably affects several parameters related to heart disease risk, including lowering total and LDL cholesterol, reducing inflammation, lowering blood pressure, and reducing plaque formation. Recent research suggests that adding black cumin seed oil to a regimen of either omega-3 fatty acids (fish oil) or astaxanthin can enhance the anti-inflammatory and anti-oxidant benefits above and beyond simply an additive effect.

Palm Fruit Extract

Palm fruits grow in tropical regions around the world such as Malaysia, Indonesia, Nigeria, and recently in Mexico. Typically grown for its oil content, palm fruit also contains a highly unique collection of water-soluble polyphenols (shikimic acid and several derivatives) that support optimal total cardiac output, a decreased workload or pressure on the heart, and a reduction of oxidative and inflammatory stress to help preserve mental wellness. Preclinical research in animals has demonstrated the potent antioxidant properties of palm fruit bioactives (PFBs), which include the upregulation of specific phase II detoxifying enzymes, a decrease in levels of reactive oxygen species, and an increase in the level of intracellular glutathione and heme oxygenase, both of which can profoundly protect delicate heart and brain cells from cellular stress. The beta-amyloid peptide appears to play a key role in the decrease of brain function over time, eventually leading to dementia and Alzheimer's disease. In several preclinical research studies in animals, PFB has been shown to inhibit beta-amyloid aggregation, potentially protecting the brain from age-induced damage. PFB has also been shown to increase levels of nitric oxide synthase and higher levels of nitric oxide, leading to vasodilation of blood vessels; improved oxygen delivery to the heart, muscles, and brain; and overall improvements in physical performance and mental fitness. Recent clinical trials on PFB supplementation in moderately stressed subjects have shown a dramatic increase in oxidation-reduction potential, suggesting not only that PFB can directly protect cells from stress, but it can also enhance the internal cellular machinery that allows the cells to protect themselves. In addition, PFB supplementation resulted in a 22 percent improvement in levels of BDNF, a major contributor to neuronal plasticity, and with improved mood and memory as well as substantial improvements in psychological mood state (50 percent lower depression indices and 25 percent lower fatigue indices), suggesting a dual heart-brain benefit from the collection of polyphenols in PFB.

Mango Leaf Extract

Mango leaf extract has a long history of use in tropical areas where mangoes are grown as a "body and brain tonic" to elevate mental and physical energy levels. Recently, mango leaf extracts have been shown to be high in anti-inflammatory compounds called xanthones. These high-xanthone extracts have been studied in seven clinical trials—showing enhanced mental energy (cognitive performance, brain electrophysiology, and reaction time) and improved sports performance (higher power output, reduced fatigue, and accelerated post exercise recovery).

Lychee Fruit Extract

Lychee fruit extract is extremely rich in highly-absorbed polyphenols, including catechin monomers and proanthocyanidin oligomers, and has been shown in more than two dozen clinical trials to reduce body weight, waist circumference (by more than an inch; 3 cm), and visceral (belly) fat by 12 percent (compared to baseline and placebo over 10 weeks). In addition, lychee fruit extract has also been shown to reduce stress hormones (cortisol) and inflammatory cytokines (IL-6 and IL-1beta) in a

4-week randomized controlled trial—and after 12 weeks has been shown to improve skin tone, texture, smoothness, and resiliency (reduction in appearance of freckles/blemishes and wrinkle length/depth).

Supplements to Support the Gut-Heart-Brain Axis

When it comes to supplementing our "axis," it is very easy to get confused because of the complex and overlapping nature of how communication signals move across the different parts of our axis to and from our gut and brain and heart. As discussed in chapter 4, our axis encompasses our nervous system (nerves), endocrine system (hormones), and circulatory system (blood) and involves hundreds of signaling molecules, such as neurotransmitters, fatty acids, hormones, endocannabinoids, and many others. Perhaps the most important (and modifiable) pathway in our entire axis is our immune system, which science is increasingly suggesting should be thought of as a "communication organ" within the body—sort of a cellular "Pony Express" to pick up and deliver messages from one part of the body to another.

As I write these words during the COVID-19 pandemic and the global quarantines of 2020, millions of people are concerned about both their mental fitness and their immune function—and hardly any of them fully grasp how interconnected and dependent each is on the other.

Unfortunately, most of us think about our immune system only when it is too late—after we become infected and get sick. At that point, we feel terrible mentally and physically, and we think we need to "stimulate" our immune system to help us feel better, but this is actually not the best approach. Overstimulation of our immune system can be just as bad or worse than having a suppressed or underactive immune system. An underactive immune system certainly puts us at a higher risk for viral infections (such as colds, flus, and COVID-19), for bacterial infections (such as foodborne illnesses related to *Salmonella* in chicken and *E. coli* in hamburgers), and even for certain types of cancer, because these are all factors that a properly tuned immune system should be looking out for, identifying, and fighting before any one of them becomes a problem. On the flip side, an overactive immune system, especially if it doesn't have an "enemy" to attack (such as a virus, bacteria, or cancer), is likely to start attacking you—which is what we see in allergies, food intolerances, and autoimmune diseases, such as rheumatoid arthritis, lupus, type 1 diabetes, Crohn's disease, multiple sclerosis, and many others.

What we actually want from our immune system is for its activity to be "just right"—not too low or too high—so that it can quickly leap into action when it needs to, efficiently and effectively deal with the threat, and quietly go into the background as the surveillance and communication organ that it is designed to be. This is referred to as immune system "priming"—training and educating the immune system to be smart and ready but not agitated into a state where it attacks everything in sight. When we have a properly primed immune system, not only are we less likely to get sick, we are also more likely to feel well, meaning that in addition to fewer colds and flus and fewer allergies and food intolerances, we actually have heightened levels of psychological vigor (physical energy + mental acuity + emotional well-being).

Unfortunately, while there might be a lot of supplements on the market that claim to "stimulate" the immune system (echinacea, elderberry, high doses of zinc and vitamin C, and various others), there are relatively few that have been clinically validated for a true priming effect. Luckily, the few that have been studied show a high degree of safety and effectiveness—so while there are not a lot of choices, those that are available are very good.

Vitamin D

You might think of vitamin D as being "good for strong bones" and helping prevent osteoporosis—and that is true, because it helps the body absorb calcium from the diet. The more recent and exciting news is that vitamin D can help reduce the risk of a wide range of diseases, including diabetes, heart attacks, high blood pressure, chronic pain, multiple sclerosis, depression, stroke, rheumatoid arthritis, and cancers of the lung, prostate, kidney, esophagus, breast, ovary, stomach, and bladder. Vitamin D also acts as an immune system modulator (priming versus stimulating) helping to prevent excessive expression of inflammatory cytokines and increasing the oxidative-burst potential of macrophages (cells that are part of the immune system's immediate activation of the innate immune system). Scientific evidence also suggests that vitamin D deficiencies are linked to immune-related conditions, including autism and asthma. For example, the seasonal vitamin D deficiency that spikes during the winter months (when sun exposure is reduced) has been associated with not only mood problems such as seasonal affective disorder but also with immune system dysfunction such as multiple sclerosis, type 1 diabetes, rheumatoid arthritis, and autoimmune thyroid disease. Many scientists have even suggested that the vitamin D deficiency that comes with the winter months may be the seasonal trigger for influenza outbreaks around the world.

Very few foods are good sources of vitamin D, but you can get some in fortified dairy products and breakfast cereals, fatty fish, and egg yolks. Cod-liver oil is a good source of vitamin D but also tends to contain too much vitamin A, which can interfere with the absorption and activity of vitamin D in the body. This makes vitamin D supplementation almost mandatory for anyone who wants better mental fitness or a stronger immune system or, ideally, both. The two forms of vitamin D found in dietary supplements are D-2 (ergocalciferol) and D-3 (cholecalciferol), with D-3 being the preferred form because it is chemically equivalent to the form of vitamin D naturally produced by the body and is two to three times more effective than the D-2 form at raising blood levels of vitamin D. A daily dose of 2,000 IU of vitamin D-3 would be expected to raise blood levels by 20 ng/mL, which is about the amount of "deficiency" that the average person might expect to have (especially during the winter months in a northern-latitude city in the United States). I live in Utah, a pretty sunny state, so during the summer months I take 1,000 IU every day, while in the snowier winter months I take 5,000 IU on a daily basis.

Beta-glucan

Beta-glucan is a generic term for "beta-1,3-linked polyglucose," which is a polysaccharide (basically a long chain of sugar molecules) found in the cell walls of yeast cells and some plants. Purified beta-glucan (derived from yeast) is known to help the immune system to better fight off infections, cold and flu viruses, and cancer and tumors. When the immune system is out of balance (high or low), it not only fails to protect the body from invading pathogens (bacteria and viruses) but can even attack it, mistaking the body's own cells for dangerous pathogens, resulting in oxidative and inflammatory autoimmune diseases, such as lupus and rheumatoid arthritis. Allergies can result when the immune system is "overactive" and mistakes an innocuous and harmless particle (such as pollen or cat dander) for an invading pathogen. Another side effect of an immune system that is out of balance is chronic low-grade inflammation, which can increase risks for cancer and heart disease and other chronic diseases related to elevated inflammation, such as depression. Beta-glucan supplements are one of the most well-researched approaches to priming the immune system and improving mental fitness (psychological vigor) by controlling and "guiding" the activity of the innate immune system.

Beta-glucans can be found in the cell walls of bacteria, fungi, yeasts, algae, lichens, and plants such as oats and barley. They act as immune-modulator agents, meaning they trigger a cascade of events that help regulate the immune system, making it more efficient. Specifically, beta-glucans stimulate the activity of macrophages, which are versatile immune cells that ingest and demolish invading pathogens and stimulate other immune cells to attack. Macrophages also release cytokines, chemicals that when secreted enable the immune cells to communicate with one another. In addition, beta-glucans stimulate lethal white blood cells (lymphocytes and natural killer cells) that bind to tumors or viruses, releasing antitumor and antiviral chemicals. Beta-glucan derived from yeast cell walls (*Saccharomyces cerevisiae*) has been shown to be particularly effective in priming immune function and activating key innate immune cells, enhancing immune system function, boosting psychological vigor, and elevating overall well-being.

Fucoidan

A slightly different type of polysaccharide (long chain of natural sugars) that can be complementary to beta-glucan is extracted from three types of brown seaweed: *Cladosiphon okamuranus, Laminaria japonica,* and *Undaria pinnatifida.* These species of seaweed contain high levels of fucoidan (a sulfated polysaccharide) shown to promote healthy immune system modulation, improved cell-to-cell communication, and superior tissue maintenance. Fucoidan may also directly improve gastric activity and ease a range of GI discomfort symptoms, including bloating, heartburn, stomachache, and other postprandial (after eating) symptoms.

Alpha-Glucan

Yet another slightly different polysaccharide structure is seen with the alpha-glucans that can be extracted from mushrooms such as maitake, shiitake, button, chaga, and others. Mushrooms in general and alpha-glucans specifically have demonstrated an ability to enhance a wide range of immune system functions. One very specialized alpha-glucan called active hexose correlated compound (AHCC) is a "cultured mycelium extract" from shiitake mushrooms. This means that rather than the alpha-glucans being extracted from the above-ground portion of the mushroom (the "fruiting body"), these alpha-glucans are extracted from the underground mycelium (the roots or nervous system of the mushroom). AHCC is manufactured through an extended lipid culturing process that results in incredibly unique active components that are supported by over thirty human clinical studies showing support for both innate and adaptive immune responses. Studies have shown that AHCC can reduce stress hormone exposure, improve mood and energy levels in people suffering from chronic fatigue, and stimulate the activity of several types of immune cells, including natural killer cells (involved in the defense against viral infections and cancer cells) and dendritic cells (that regulate immune response between the innate and adaptive systems). AHCC is also directly beneficial for gut health, with research demonstrating its capacity to reduce intestinal inflammation and to favor the development of a healthy gut microbiome with more *Bifidobacterium* and less *Clostridium* and *E.coli*.

Multivitamins

It almost goes without saying that taking a general multivitamin and mineral supplement is a good idea for anybody who is under stress, maintains a hectic lifestyle, or wants to improve their mental fitness. Every energy-related reaction that takes place in the body, especially those involved in the stress response, relies in one way or another on vitamins and minerals as "cofactors" to make the reactions go. For example, B-complex vitamins are needed to metabolize protein and carbohydrates. Chromium is likewise involved in handling carbohydrates. Magnesium and calcium are needed for proper muscle contraction. Zinc and copper are required as enzyme cofactors in nearly three hundred separate reactions. Iron is needed to help shuttle oxygen in the blood. The list goes on and on. It is fairly well accepted across the global scientific community that subclinical or marginal deficiencies of essential micronutrients—especially the B-complex vitamins, vitamin D, magnesium, and omega-3 fatty acids—can lead to psychological and physiological symptoms that are related to stress and poor mental fitness. This is why I recommend a well-balanced multivitamin and a separate omega-3 supplement for everyone. When looking for a balanced multivitamin/mineral supplement, you will find that there are hundreds and hundreds of offerings, each with their particular pros and cons. Make sure that whichever one you choose has at least 100 percent of the daily value for the following nutrients crucial to supporting the entire gut-heart-brain axis:

Vitamin B6

Tryptophan is an essential amino acid that helps regulate nervous system activity related to relaxation and sleep. Vitamin B6 converts a small amount of the tryptophan in your body to serotonin (our key "happiness" neurotransmitter) and then to melatonin (our primary "sleep hormone").

Without an adequate amount of vitamin B6 in your diet, your body's metabolism of tryptophan may be disturbed. This may limit the amount of serotonin and melatonin in your body, potentially leading to mood disturbances, disrupted sleep patterns, and insomnia.

Vitamin B12

Cobalamin, or vitamin B12, is important for a number of essential processes in the body, including the production of DNA and RNA, the regulation of blood cell formation, and the maintenance of neurons. Vitamin B12 deficiency results in anemia, nerve damage, depression, memory impairment, irritability, psychosis, personality changes, and other psychological symptoms because the vitamin is required for the formation of neurotransmitters such as serotonin and dopamine. These symptoms are further worsened when folate deficiency is also present. Therefore, vitamin B12 supplementation can improve sleep, stress regulation, energy levels, and overall mood by providing relief for depression and by preventing damage to nerve cells in the brain.

Niacin

Also known as vitamin B3, niacin is vital for overall brain performance, including mood, sleep patterns, and neuron metabolism. Low niacin levels disrupt the firing of brain neurons and, therefore, affects our mood, memory, and sleep-wake cycle. Niacin is often thought of as an "energy" vitamin, but it is equally considered to be a "relaxation and mood" vitamin due to its participation in a wide array of metabolic reactions.

Folic Acid

Folic acid, also known as vitamin B9, is another "multifunctional" nutrient, with roles in regulating heartbeat, nerve function, mental focus, memory, and mood. These symptoms can affect sleep either directly or indirectly.

Vitamin C

Vitamin C, also known as ascorbic acid, is essential for serotonin production. Studies show that a lack of vitamin C may cause mood problems as well as shorter and nonrestorative sleep. Vitamin C is also required to produce dopamine, norepinephrine, and epinephrine—neurotransmitters that boost physical and mental energy and feelings of reward and satisfaction.

Vitamin D

Vitamin D is involved in hundreds of metabolic reactions related to neurotransmitter metabolism, overall mood, and mental function, including a wide range of processes that help to regulate immune function (a crucial portion of the "axis" in our gut-heart-brain axis). Lack of vitamin D is associated with the depression symptoms that come with seasonal affective disorder, and vitamin D supplements (as well as sunlight exposure) can be effective in restoring normal metabolism and thus boosting mood and mental fitness.

Magnesium

Sufficient levels of magnesium are required to stimulate melatonin synthesis and maintain optimal nerve transmission. Not only can magnesium help you get to sleep, but it plays a part in helping you achieve deep and restful sleep as well. Magnesium deficiency has been shown to result in sleep patterns that were light and restless—an effect that is partially due to magnesium's influence in "calming" the nervous system.

Zinc

Zinc plays an essential role in neurotransmitter function and helps maintain cognition, due to its involvement in both melatonin and dopamine metabolism.

Whew!

You made it through the longest chapter in the book—congratulations. I hope it gives you a perspective that there is a long menu of very safe, very effective options to nourish our entire gut-heart-brain axis with targeted dietary supplementation. But as I have been saying from the very beginning, they are each just one piece of the puzzle. It is up to each and every one of us to find the right pieces that click together in the right pattern to improve our mental fitness in the way(s) that are most aligned with where we are now and where we want to be in the future. For some of us, that might mean that we want to "feel better" by lowering our stress levels. For others, it might mean not lowering stress at all but instead increasing resilience. For still others, it might be some combination of better sleep plus a sharper mind plus fewer (or more) trips to the bathroom. The focus should be less on the individual supplements or isolated components and more on designing the holistic regimen and philosophy—the system and journey—that you can follow on a regular basis to take your mental fitness to whatever level you desire.

CHAPTER 10

THE TROJAN HORSE:
HOW MENTAL FITNESS
DRIVES PHYSICAL HEALTH

At this point in the book, you may have already figured out the "end-ing," which essentially is this: by improving our mental fitness, we can also improve our physical health and even our longevity.

This is what I often refer to as the "Trojan Horse of Health," which in a sense "tricks" us into focusing on "feeling better" with superior mental fitness (less stress, better mood, sharper focus, greater energy, and higher resilience), while at the same time we're moving ourselves step-by-step toward better physical health (lower body fat, improved heart health, consistent blood sugar balance, better mobility, and less physical pain).

I've used this "feel better first" approach for nearly two decades to help people feel good "now" (within hours to days to weeks) while they are getting healthier "later" (across weeks to months to years), and it has worked wonders to help reverse obesity, diabetes, dementia, arthritis, chronic fatigue, fibromyalgia, depression, anxiety, PTSD (post-traumatic stress disorder), ADHD (attention-deficit hyperactivity disorder), IBS (irritable bowel syndrome), and chronic pain.

Remember that the fable of the Trojan Horse is a story from Greek mythology, where Odysseus and a small team of elite soldiers hide them-selves inside a huge wooden horse, which was the symbol of the Trojans and the city of Troy. As the story goes, after ten unsuccessful years of besieging the city of Troy, the Greek army gave up and sailed home, leaving a "peace offering" of the giant horse as a symbol of Troy's victory. Unknown to the Trojans, who pulled the horse within the city walls, the Greek army sailed back under cover of darkness and were greeted by Odysseus and his men who had sneaked out of the horse to open the gates from the inside, resulting in the fall of Troy.

As a metaphor, a "Trojan Horse" has come to describe a variety of strategies for diverting focus away from one thing and toward another. In our case, we avert our focus on "getting healthier" (which is often a long and difficult process) toward the more compelling and immediate benefit of "feeling better" (which is often quicker and easier).

Why Mental Fitness Fuels Physical Health

For people who suffer from depression or anxiety, a companion diagnosis with a physical health condition is almost assured. In medical lingo, we refer to the co-occurrence of different diseases as "comorbid" conditions—and it is more common than not to see depression/pain, anxiety/IBS, and burnout/heart disease being diagnosed as a package deal. Far from being "bad luck," recent research indicates quite clearly that this type of dual diagnosis is, in fact, quite closely connected through the gut-heart-brain axis.

Doctors have certainly observed the links between mental and physical health problems for centuries, but the association was typically chalked up to behavioral factors. For example, depressed people are less likely to take their medications or practice healthy habits, so they get sicker. Sick people experience pain and impaired function, which affects their emotional state: think about someone with chronic back pain, dealing with unrelenting discomfort day in and day out, and it's not surprising to see higher rates of depression. However, advances in biochemistry, physiology, psychology, and genomics have enabled us to tease out the underlying factors across the gut-heart-brain axis that are actually at the root of the mind/body or mental/physical relationship.

To illustrate how the mind-body connection actually belies a seemingly "body-only" condition, let us consider psoriasis and eczema, which are autoimmune conditions that cause red patches and flaky scales on the skin. Depression and stress, as well as microbiome imbalances, are common among people with these skin conditions, who often deal with discomfort and the social stigma related to their condition.

Several researchers have found that psoriasis patients are more likely to develop depression, and those with depression are more likely to also develop psoriatic arthritis (a complication that involves inflammation of the joints). Even after controlling for differences in diet quality, exercise levels, and body weight, the increased risk of progression from body (skin rash) to brain (depression) and back to body (arthritis) persisted, suggesting that there is an underlying root cause or causes that are common to what might first appear to be different conditions.

As we have covered in previous chapters, research has linked depression and other mental fitness problems with an increased risk of conditions like stroke, diabetes, and rheumatoid arthritis, as well as a strong predictor of heart disease (even stronger than other well-known risk factors like obesity and high cholesterol).

At this point of the book, all of this might make sense and you might be thinking of inflammation or cortisol or leaky gut or microbiome dysbiosis or any one of the many potential targets across the gut-heart-brain axis that we have discussed in the previous chapters. But there is an important caveat that we need to keep in mind: these mind/body conditions are the very definition of "multi-factorial" problems, and as such, they require a multi-factorial solution to help us feel and perform at our best.

Trying to solve depression or other mental fitness problems with "only" medication or "only" talk therapy (or even a combination of both) is a fool's errand. We have ample scientific and anecdotal evidence that such limited approaches barely scratch the surface in terms of optimizing mental fitness. Rather, we need to recognize that the more comprehensive and holistic we can get with our lifestyle interventions, the more effective we can be in helping people reach their peak potential. This is why our expanded understanding of the gut-heart-brain axis is so important: restoring balance across as many aspects of it as possible can help us to feel better in the short term, while we are improving health and reducing the risk of future problems in the long term.

Mental Pain and Physical Pain: Two Sides of the Same Coin

The artificial distinction in modern medicine between the mind and the body is slowly starting to erode in the wake of a wide range of research studies showing a clear and compelling bi-directional relationship between body pain and emotional distress. It is now quite clear that the chronic health conditions that have fatigue and pain as defining factors are significant risk factors for future development of psychological problems such as depression, anxiety, and burnout. The opposite is also true: individuals with psychological problems (particularly depression) tend to be at higher risk for chronic health problems including obesity, diabetes, heart disease, irritable bowel syndrome, and fibromyalgia. Even when we are not technically dealing with "diseases" of the body and mind, it is quite clear that struggling with physical or mental symptoms on any level can be expected to lead to "quality of life" issues such as sleep disturbances, impaired work/school performance, and general barriers to social functioning.

Even though we know quite clearly that mental pain and physical pain are closely linked, we often lack a clear understanding of why or how this linkage exists. As discussed in earlier chapters, we know that the gut has its own nervous system (the ENS, or enteric nervous system) that links to the brain (the CNS, or central nervous system) via the hypothalamic-pituitary-adrenal axis. Chronic stimulation of the HPA axis (stress) is thought to sensitize the CNS and ENS so signals are amplified, meaning that pain sensations in the body are more painful and pain sensations in the mind are more depressing. In a similar fashion, psychological distress can also undermine immune system function and increase inflammatory signaling, thereby intensifying the effects of physical illness. In fact, for many years, many scientists thought that chronic inflammation was at the root of virtually every human health malady, including heart disease and depression.

A more nuanced appraisal of the most recent science suggests that, while inflammation is certainly an important underlying factor, the regulation of inflammation by the immune system and its orchestration by the gut microbiome may be even more deeply rooted as the ultimate underlying cause of the mind/body linkage. This is not to say that the microbiome is our new scientific silver bullet, and that all we have to do is fix our microbiome and we will be fine. Rather, it is to emphasize the point that there are multiple "levels" at which we can use natural therapies in a holistic, multi-factorial "systems approach" to restore balance comprehensively across the entire gut-heart-brain axis in order to optimize mental fitness and physical health.

How Old is Your Gut?

In addition to the prominent role the microbiome plays when it comes to determining our mental fitness, it is emerging as a key player in aging and longevity as well. This means that while we are modulating microbiome balance to "feel better now" with better mood, sharper focus, higher energy, and better resilience, we may also be helping ourselves "age better later" and live longer with a reduced risk of chronic age-related diseases.

Over a century ago, Élie Metchnikoff proposed that the majority of age-related health problems were the result of chronic, systemic inflammation caused by increased colon permeability—something that we understand today as "leaky gut," "endotoxemia," and "inflamm-aging"—all of which are now identified by modern scientific studies as prominent underlying causes of human aging.

In general, healthy adults tend to have high levels of bacteria from two major phyla: Bacteroidetes, which are involved in the metabolism of fiber, a highly complex carbohydrate, and Firmicutes, which tend to thrive on simple carbohydrates such as sugar. Each phyla participates in myriad other aspects of metabolism, but research has shown that the ratio between them (the "F/B ratio") can be used as an important indicator of microbiome balance and overall health. For example, a higher F/B ratio (higher Firmicutes and/or lower Bacteroidetes) is associated with diabetes, weight gain, and overall microbiome imbalance (dysbiosis), while a lower F/B ratio is associated with improved metabolism and more successful aging.

Older people also generally have a lower diversity of bacteria in their microbiome, with particular reductions in "good" bacterial species such as *Bifidobacterium* and *Lactobacillus* and increases in *E. coli* and Enterobacteria (both of which can damage the gut lining and lead to leaky gut). Interestingly, studies in centenarians (people over 100 years of age) and supercentenarians (those over 110) have shown particularly high levels of *Bifidobacteria* (which produce short-chain fatty acids)—and supplementing these bacteria has increased longevity in studies of worms, flies, and mice—so the potential promise for humans could be on the horizon.

Because of the close link between our gut microbiome and our immune system function, the underlying mechanism of the microbiome/aging relationship might be that a reduced microbiome diversity (dysbiosis) leads to a certain level of immune system suppression, and thus a greater risk for infection, cancer proliferation, inflammatory cellular damage, and poor tissue repair.

A number of human aging studies have shown a decline in SCFA levels, particularly butyrate, which is a primary energy source for enterocytes, the cells lining our gut. So, again, we see strong relationships between what is happening in our gut and how the rest of the body performs. As you might imagine, centenarians also have a higher level of SCFAs, which is a direct result of their higher levels of butyrate-producing bacteria (*Bifidobacteria*).

This is Your Brain on a Healthy Lifestyle

We have already covered how healthy lifestyle choices such as regular physical activity, balanced diet, and cognitive engagement are key factors in maintaining mental fitness—how you feel and perform right now—but they are also just as important for how well we age in the future.

Physical activity and diet modulate common pathways throughout the mind and body, including neuron signaling, inflammation, stress response, antioxidant defenses, and blood sugar balance, among many others. Cognitive engagement such as learning a new task like playing an instrument or speaking a new language, completing a puzzle, or traveling to a new destination can enhance the "reserves" of our brain, directly reducing our risk for dementia and indirectly improving our stress resilience through an improvement in our cognitive flexibility and strategic problem solving. The best news of all is that combining physical activity with proper diet and cognitive tasks amplifies the mind/body benefits so we learn better and faster and age more slowly in every tissue system across our gut-brain-heart axis.

These effects seem to be even more pronounced when they occur in mid-life when lifestyle and environmental stressors tend to be at their peak. For example, the ability of a proper lifestyle to "buffer" the detrimental effects of stress has been demonstrated in multiple studies of the brain (such as how mindfulness meditation enhances BDNF levels and stimulates brain plasticity); the heart (such as how both strength and endurance exercise increase heart rate variability and promote mind/body resilience); the gut (such as how polyphenols in fruits/vegetables restore microbiome balance and gut integrity); and many aspects of the axis (such as reducing inflammation and priming the immune system to prevent the aging of the immune system known as "immune-senescence").

The Brain-Body-Biome Connection

Perhaps the most consistent and demonstrable connection between the mind and body is the linkage of obesity and depression. Globally, more than 1.9 billion people struggle with their weight, while depression and anxiety affect nearly 700 million.

My research group has conducted a series of clinical trials over several years to investigate how effectively we could manage both brain and body outcomes by using combinations of probiotics, prebiotics, postbiotics, and phytonutrients to modulate microbiome balance. We have presented our data at numerous scientific conferences around the world and published our results in several peer-reviewed scientific journals (see references and visit MentalFitness.tv for ongoing updates).

Our multi-year project encompasses a series of coordinated research trials intended to tease out the links between gut-brain axis function and mental wellness (Study 1); between the heart-brain axis and mental wellness (Study 2); and between mental wellness and physical health (Study 3). An overarching theme between studies and across the entire project has been that a wide range of natural ingredients (probiotics, prebiotics, postbiotics, phytonutrients, and herbal extracts) can help to restore balance within the interconnected gut-heart-brain axis to dramatically and dynamically improve mental wellness parameters.

➤ Study 1 (Gut-Brain Axis) assessed microbiome parameters (e.g., *Lactobacillus, Bifidobacterium, Akkermansia,* etc.) and correlated those levels to psychological outcomes (e.g., depression, anxiety, stress).

➤ Study 2 (Heart-Brain Axis) assessed heart efficiency (heart rate variability) and correlated those levels with mental/physical energy parameters (e.g., energy, focus, vigor).

➤ Study 3 (Mental/Physical Health) showed how improvements in mental wellness (brain), brought about by balancing gut and heart parameters, were also linked to improvements in physical health (blood glucose, cholesterol, cardiac risk, cortisol).

We have shown—and published in a series of peer-reviewed scientific journal articles—that specific nutritional ingredients can deliver meaningful improvements in overall well-being and psychological mood states through well-defined mechanisms of action including improved microbiome balance, lowered inflammation, primed immune function, increased heart rate variability, improved cardiac risk profiles, balanced blood sugar, and reduced stress hormones.

These individual studies—and the overall project—demonstrate that natural nutritional interventions very well may be the solution to one of our most pressing global epidemics, as well as being one that is open and accessible to all without the high cost, marginal benefits, and severe side effects of existing synthetic options.

Across these studies, we confirmed that targeted nutritional interventions could reliably, predictably, and simultaneously improve both mental wellness and physical health. Our studies are ongoing in order to expand our understanding of using natural nutritional interventions to move people from "bad" to "wellness" and further toward "optimized and flourishing."

Final Words

The basic truth with which we began this book—and which bears repeating here as we come to a close—is that the biggest health problems today are not physical ailments such as heart disease, cancer, and diabetes, but rather mental conditions like depression, anxiety, chronic fatigue, sleep deprivation, and everyday stress.

When we're stressed, we're more likely to crave junk food and store belly fat, but when we're resilient, we don't succumb to stress-eating and we make better dietary choices.

When we're tired, we're less likely to exercise or meditate, but when we have good sleep quality and metabolism, we have abundant energy levels that can fuel our lifestyle.

When we're depressed, we're less likely to take care of ourselves or interact positively with others, but when we have a good mood, we're more likely to love ourselves and apply that love to others.

It's no overstatement to say that "mental wellness" is, by any measure, the most compelling growth opportunity within pharmaceutical and biotech industry, within the health-care industry (often referred to disparagingly as the "disease-care" industry), within the broader wellness spa industry, and within the natural products industry, which encompasses functional foods, dietary supplements, and numerous aspects of the nutrition and healthier eating sectors. These are just some of the reasons that I started a Certified Mental Wellness Coach program to educate and train people to help others improve their mental fitness.

I want to end this chapter, and the book, by emphasizing that everything we have covered in *Mental Fitness* is not just scientifically validated and "true," but that it is all very much "do-able" within the context of your busy life. I love the science, but what I love even more is the ability to *apply* the science in an actual day-to-day setting. That is what matters most in terms of delivering real benefits to real people.

As I present these and other results at scientific conferences all over the globe, and as I interact with researchers and clinicians with different expertise across varied health disciplines, it is becoming increasingly clear that both psychological problems and physical ailments are reaching epidemic levels, and there is an urgent need for us to do something different.

Our ancient bodies and minds have clearly been outpaced in their evolution by our more rapidly advancing modern world, and we are all paying the price in terms of our mental fitness and physical health. At no other time in human history has there been as much depression, anxiety, burnout, heart disease, cancer, diabetes, chronic pain, and everyday stress and tension as there is today. Likewise, we have been awash for decades in synthetic pharmaceuticals intended to "treat" these modern ailments, yet the incidence of disease continues unabated and affects kids and teens just as much—if not more—than it does adults.

I believe that *Mental Fitness* can be an important part of our road map toward the multi-factorial approach that we need to restore balance across our three brains and entire gut-heart-brain axis. Only by applying a multi-factorial solution to our global multi-factorial problem can we hope to achieve our peak individual potential in this one life that we all have to live.

I hope you take the opportunity to apply some of the principles from this book in your own life so that you may maximize both your own mental fitness and the lives of those around you.

REFERENCES

Abildgaard, A. et al. (2017).Probiotic treatment reduces depressive-like behaviour in rats independently of diet. *Psychoneuroendocrinology* 79:40–48. doi:10.1016/j.psyneuen.2017.02.014.

Ait-Belgnaoui, A. et. al. (2018). Bifidobacterium longum and Lactobacillus helveticus Synergistically Suppress Stress-related Visceral Hypersensitivity Through Hypothalamic-Pituitary-Adrenal Axis Modulation. *J Neurogastroenterol Motil* 24(1):138–146. doi: 10.5056/jnm16167.

Akbaraly, T. N. et al. (2009). Dietary pattern and depressive symptoms in middle age. *Br J Psychiatry* 195(5):408–13.

Anhe, F. F. et al. (2015). A polyphenol-rich cranberry extract protects from diet-induced obesity, insulin resistance and intestinal inflammation in association with increased Akkermansia spp. population in the gut microbiota of mice. *Gut* 64(6):872–83.

Attuquayefio, T. and R. J. Stevenson (2015). A systematic review of longer-term dietary interventions on human cognitive function: Emerging patterns and future directions. *Appetite* 95:554–70.

Beilharz, J. E. et al. (2015). Diet-Induced Cognitive Deficits: The Role of Fat and Sugar, Potential Mechanisms and Nutritional Interventions. *Nutrients* 7(8):6719–6738.

Berk, M. et al. (2013). So depression is an inflammatory disease, but where does the inflammation come from? *BMC Medicine* 11:200.

Biesiekierski, J. R. et al. (2011). Gluten causes gastrointestinal symptoms in subjects without celiac disease: a double-blind randomized placebo-controlled trial. *Am J Gastroenterol* 106(3):508–14.

Biesiekierski, J. R. et al. (2013). No effects of gluten in patients with self-reported non-celiac gluten sensitivity after dietary reduction of fermentable, poorly absorbed, short-chain carbohydrates. *Gastroenterology* 145(2):320–8.

Bilbo, S. D. and V. Tsang (2010). Enduring consequences of maternal obesity for brain inflammation and behavior of offspring. *FASEB J* 24(6):2104–15.

Boets, E. et al. (2017). Systemic availability and metabolism of colonic-derived short-chain fatty acids in healthy subjects: a stable isotope study. *J Physiol* 15;595(2):541–555. doi:10.1113/JP272613. Epub 2016 Sep 18.

Bookheimer , S. Y. et al. (2013). Pomegranate juice augments memory and FMRI activity in middle-aged and older adults with mild memory complaints. *Evid Based Complement Alternat Med* 2013:946298. doi:10.1155/2013/946298. Epub 2013 Jul 22.

Borge, T. C. et al. (2017). The importance of maternal diet quality during pregnancy on cognitive and behavioural outcomes in children: a systematic review and meta-analysis. *BMJ Open* 7(9):e016777.

Brietzke, E. et al. (2018). Gluten related illnesses and severe mental disorders: a comprehensive review. *Neurosci Biobehav Rev* 84:368–75.

Castaner, O. et al. (2018). The Gut Microbiome Profile in Obesity: A Systematic Review. *Int J Endocrinol* 2018;2018:4095789. doi:10.1155/2018/4095789.

Chassaing, B. et al. (2015). Dietary emulsifiers impact the mouse gut microbiota promoting colitis and metabolic syndrome. *Nature* 519(7541):92–6.

Chatterton, M. L. et al. (2018). Economic evaluation of a dietary intervention for adults with major depression (the 'SMILES' trial). *BMC Public Health* 18(1):599.

Cherbuin, N. et al. (2012). Higher normal fasting plasma glucose is associated with hippocampal atrophy: The PATH Study. *Neurology* 79(10):1019–26.

Chovanová, Z. et al. (2006). Effect of polyphenolic extract, Pycnogenol, on the level of 8-oxoguanine in children suffering from attention deficit/hyperactivity disorder. *Free Radic Res* 40(9):1003–10. doi:10.1080/10715760600824902.

Christ, A. et al. (2018). Western Diet Triggers NLRP3-Dependent Innate Immune Reprogramming. *Cell* 172(1–2):162–75 e114.

Clayton, P. and J. Rowbotham (2009). How the mid-Victorians worked, ate and died. *Int J Environ Res Public Health* 6(3):1235–53.

Cotillard, A. et al. (2013). Dietary intervention impact on gut microbial gene richness [published correction appears in *Nature*. 502(7472)580]. *Nature* 500(7464):585–588. doi:10.1038/nature12480.

Croll, P. H. et al. (2018). Better diet quality relates to larger brain tissue volumes: The Rotterdam Study. *Neurology* 90(24):e2166–73.

Curtis, J. et al. (2016). Evaluating an individualized lifestyle and life skills intervention to prevent antipsychotic-induced weight gain in first-episode psychosis. *Early Interv Psychiatry* 10(3):267–76.

Dai, X. et al. (2015). Consuming Lentinula edodes (Shiitake) Mushrooms Daily Improves Human Immunity: A Randomized Dietary Intervention in Healthy Young Adults. *J Am Coll Nutr* 34(6):478–87. doi:10.1080/07315724.2014.950391. Epub 2015 Apr 11.

Dai, Z. et al. (2017). Effects of α-Galactooligosaccharides from Chickpeas on

High-Fat-Diet-Induced Metabolic Syndrome in Mice. *J Agric Food Chem* 65(15):3160–3166. doi:10.1021/acs.jafc.7b00489. Epub 2017 Apr 6.

Davison, G. et al. (2016). Zinc carnosine works with bovine colostrum in truncating heavy exercise-induced increase in gut permeability in healthy volunteers. *Am J Clin Nutr* 104(2):526–36. doi:10.3945/ajcn.116.134403. Epub 2016 Jun 29.

Desrosiers, T. A. et al. (2018). Low carbohydrate diets may increase risk of neural tube defects. *Birth Defects Res* 110(11):901–09.

Devaraj, S. et al. (2002). Supplementation with a pine bark extract rich in polyphenols increases plasma antioxidant capacity and alters the plasma lipoprotein profile. *Lipids* 37(10):931–4. doi:10.1007/s11745-006-0982-3.

Devkota, S. et al. (2012). Dietary-fat-induced taurocholic acid promotes pathobiont expansion and colitis in Il10-/-mice. *Nature* 487(7405):104–8.

Dinan, T.G. et al (2017). Psychobiotics: a novel class of psychotropic. *Biol Psychiatry* 74(10):720–726. doi:10.1016/j.biopsych.2013.05.001.

Dipnall, J. F. et al. (2015). The association between dietary patterns, diabetes and depression. *J Affect Disord* 174:215–24.

Duncan, S. H. et al. (2007). Reduced dietary intake of carbohydrates by obese subjects results in decreased concentrations of butyrate and butyrate-producing bacteria in feces. *Appl Environ Microbiol* 73(4):1073–8.

Dvoráková, M. et al. (2006). The effect of polyphenolic extract from pine bark, Pycnogenol on the level of glutathione in children suffering from attention deficit hyperactivity disorder (ADHD). *Redox Rep* 11(4):163–72. doi:10.1179/135100006X116664.

Eskelinen, M. H. et al. (2008). Fat intake at midlife and cognitive impairment later in life: a population-based CAIDE study. *Int J Geriatr Psychiatry* 23(7):741–7.

Estruch, R. et al. (2013). Primary prevention of cardiovascular disease with a Mediterranean diet. *N Engl J Med* 368(14):1279–90.

Fardet, A. and Y. Boirie (2014). Associations between food and beverage groups and major diet-related chronic diseases: an exhaustive review of pooled/ meta-analyses and systematic reviews. *Nutr Rev* 72(12):741–62.

Foster, L. M. et al. (2011). A comprehensive post-market review of studies on a probiotic product containing Lactobacillus helveticus R0052 and Lactobacillus rhamnosus R0011. *Benef Microbes* 2(4):319–334. doi:10.3920/BM2011.0032.

Francis, H. and R. Stevenson (2013). The longer-term impacts of Western diet on human cognition and the brain. *Appetite* 63:119–28.

Fuller, R. et al. (2017). Yeast-derived β-1,3/1,6 glucan, upper respiratory tract infection and innate immunity in older adults. *Nutrition* 39–40:30–35. doi:10.1016/j.nut.2017.03.003. Epub 2017 Mar 23.

Fung, T. T. et al. (2010). Low-carbohydrate diets and all-cause and cause-specific mortality: two cohort studies. *Ann Intern Med* 153(5):289–98.

Gardner, C. D. et al. (2018). Effect of Low-Fat vs Low-Carbohydrate Diet on 12-Month Weight Loss in Overweight Adults and the Association With Genotype Pattern or Insulin Secretion: The DIETFITS Randomized Clinical Trial. *JAMA* 319(7):667–79.

Gaullier, J. M. et al. (2011). Supplementation with a soluble β-glucan exported from Shiitake medicinal mushroom, Lentinus edodes (Berk.) singer mycelium: a crossover, placebo-controlled study in healthy elderly. *Int J Med Mushrooms* 13(4):319–26. doi:10.1615/intjmedmushr.v13.i4.10.

GBD 2016 Risk Factors Collaborators (2017). Global, regional, and national incidence, prevalence, and years lived with disability for 328 diseases and injuries for 195 countries, 1990–2016: a systematic analysis for the Global Burden of Disease Study 2016. *Lancet* 390(10100):1211–59.

Giacosa, A. et al. (2015). The Effect of Ginger (Zingiber officinalis) and Artichoke (Cynara cardunculus) Extract Supplementation on Functional Dyspepsia: A Randomised, Double-Blind, and Placebo-Controlled Clinical Trial. *Evid Based Complement Alternat Med.* 2015:915087. doi:10.1155/2015/915087. Epub 2015 Apr 14.

Gibson, G. R. and M. B. Roberfroid. (1995). Dietary modulation of the human colonic microbiota: introducing the concept of prebiotics. *J Nutr* 125(6):1401–1412. doi:10.1093/jn/125.6.1401.

Grimaldi, R. et al. (2018). A prebiotic intervention study in children with autism spectrum disorders (ASDs). *Microbiome* 6(1):133. doi: 10.1186/s40168-018-0523-3.

Haast, R. A. and A. J. Kiliaan (2015). Impact of fatty acids on brain circulation, structure and function. *Prostaglandins Leukot Essent Fatty Acids* 92:3–14.

Hakkarainen, R. et al. (2003). Association of dietary amino acids with low mood. *Depress Anxiety* 18(2):89–94.

Hibberd, A. A. et al. (2019). Probiotic or synbiotic alters the gut microbiota and metabolism in a randomised controlled trial of weight management in overweight adults. *Benef Microbes* 10(2):121–135. doi:10.3920/BM2018.0028. Epub 2018 Dec 10.

Hidese, S. et al. (2019). Effects of L-Theanine Administration on Stress-Related Symptoms and Cognitive Functions in Healthy Adults: A Randomized Controlled Trial. *Nutrients* 11(10):2362. doi:10.3390/nu11102362.

Hill, C. et al. (2014). Expert consensus document. The International Scientific Association for Probiotics and Prebiotics consensus statement on the scope and appropriate use of the term probiotic. *Nat Rev Gastroenterol Hepatol* 11(8):506–514. doi:10.1038/nrgastro.2014.66.

Hong, M. et al. (2015). Probiotics (Lactobacillus rhamnosus R0011 and acidophilus R0052) reduce the expression of toll-like receptor 4 in mice with alcoholic liver disease. *PLoS One* 10(2):e0117451. doi:10.1371/journal.pone.0117451.

Indiani, C. M. D. S. P. et al. (2018). Childhood Obesity and Firmicutes/Bacteroidetes Ratio in the Gut Microbiota: A Systematic Review. *Child Obes* 14(8):501–509. doi:10.1089/chi.2018.0040.

Itagaki, M. et al. (2014). Efficacy of zinc-carnosine chelate compound, Polaprezinc, enemas in patients with ulcerative colitis. *Scand J Gastroenterol* 49(2):164–72. doi:10.3109/00365521.2013.863963. Epub 2013 Nov 29.

Ito, T. et al. (2014). Effects of enzyme-treated asparagus extract on heat shock protein 70, stress indices, and sleep in healthy adult men. *J Nutr Sci Vitaminol* (Tokyo) 60(4):283–90. doi:10.3177/jnsv.60.283.

Ito, T. et al. (2014). Enzyme-treated asparagus extract promotes expression of heat shock protein and exerts antistress effects. *J Food Sci* 79(3):H413-9. doi:10.1111/1750-3841.12371. Epub 2014 Feb 5.

Jacka, F. N. et al. (2012). Red Meat Consumption and Mood and Anxiety Disorders. *Psychother Psychosom* 81:196–8.

Jacka, F. N. et al. (2009). Association between magnesium intake and depression and anxiety in community-dwelling adults: the Hordaland Health Study. *Aust N Z J Psychiatry* 43(1):45–52.

Jacka, F. N. et al. (2010). Associations between diet quality and depressed mood in adolescents: results from the Australian Healthy Neighbourhoods Study. *Aust N Z J Psychiatry* 44(5):435–42.

Jacka, F. N. et al. (2011). A prospective study of diet quality and mental health in adolescents. *PLoS One* 6(9): e24805.

Jacka, F. N. et al. (2011). The association between habitual diet quality and the common mental disorders in community-dwelling adults: the Hordaland Health study. *Psychosom Med* 73(6):483–90.

Jacka, F. N. et al. (2013). Maternal and early postnatal nutrition and mental health of offspring by age 5 years: a prospective cohort study. *J Am Acad Child Adolesc Psychiatry* 52(10):1038–47.

Jacka, F. N. et al. (2015). Does reverse causality explain the relationship between diet and depression? *J Affect Disord* 175:248–50.

Jacka, F. N. et al. (2015). Western diet is associated with a smaller hippocampus: a longitudinal investigation. *BMC Med* 13:215.

Jacka, F. N. et al. (2017). A randomised controlled trial of dietary improvement for adults with major depression (the 'SMILES' trial). *BMC Med* 15(1):23.

Jacka, F. et al. (2010). Association of Western and traditional diets with depression and anxiety in women. *American Journal of Psychiatry* 167(3):305–11.

Kadooka, Y. et al. (2010). Regulation of abdominal adiposity by probiotics (Lactobacillus gasseri SBT2055) in adults with obese tendencies in a randomized controlled trial. *Eur J Clin Nutr* 64(6):636–643. doi:10.1038/ejcn.2010.19.

Kanoski, S. E. and T. L. Davidson (2011). Western diet consumption and cognitive impairment: links to hippocampal dysfunction and obesity. *Physiol Behav* 103(1):59–68.

Kastorini, C. M. et al. (2011). The effect of Mediterranean diet on metabolic syndrome and its components: a meta-analysis of 50 studies and 534,906 individuals. *J Am Coll Cardiol* 57(11):1299–313.

Kessler, R. C. et al. (2005). Lifetime prevalence and age-of-onset distributions of DSM-IV disorders in the National Comorbidity Survey Replication. *Arch Gen Psychiatry* 62(6):593–602.

Khalid, S. et al. (2016). Is there an association between diet and depression in children and adolescents? A systematic review. *Br J Nutr* 116(12):2097–108.

Khambadkone, S. G. et al. (2018). Nitrated meat products are associated with mania in humans and altered behavior and brain gene expression in rats. *Mol Psychiatry*.

Kim, J. et al. (2018). Lactobacillus gasseri BNR17 Supplementation Reduces the Visceral Fat Accumulation and Waist Circumference in Obese Adults: A Randomized, Double-Blind, Placebo-Controlled Trial. *J Med Food* 21(5):454–461. doi:10.1089/jmf.2017.3937.

Koliada, A. et al. (2017). Association between body mass index and Firmicutes/Bacteroidetes ratio in an adult Ukrainian population. *BMC Microbiol* 17(1):120. Published 2017 May 22. doi:10.1186/s12866-017-1027-1.

Koutsos, A. et al. (2015). Apples and cardiovascular health--is the gut microbiota a core consideration? *Nutrients* 7(6):3959–98. doi:10.3390/nu7063959.

Krakowiak, P. et al. (2012). Maternal metabolic conditions and risk for autism and other neurodevelopmental disorders. *Pediatrics* 129(5):e1121–8.

Kujawska, M. et al. (2019). Neuroprotective Effects of Pomegranate Juice against Parkinson's Disease and Presence of Ellagitannins-Derived Metabolite-Urolithin A-In the Brain. *Int J Mol Sci* 21(1):E202. doi:10.3390/ijms21010202.

Lachance, L. R. and K. McKenzie (2014). Biomarkers of gluten sensitivity in patients with non-affective psychosis: a meta-analysis. *Schizophr Res* 152(2–3):521–7.

Lam, Y. Y. et al. (2015). Effects of dietary fat profile on gut permeability and microbiota and their relationships with metabolic changes in mice. *Obesity* (Silver Spring) 23(7):1429–39.

Lazar, V. et al. (2019). Gut Microbiota, Host Organism, and Diet Trialogue in Diabetes and Obesity. *Front Nutr* 6:21. doi:10.3389/fnut.2019.00021.

Lazzini, S. et al. (2016). The effect of ginger (Zingiber officinalis) and artichoke (Cynara cardunculus) extract supplementation on gastric motility: a pilot randomized study in healthy volunteers. *Eur Rev Med Pharmacol Sci* 20(1):146–9.

Lee, S. H. et al. (2016). Is increased antidepressant exposure a contributory factor to the obesity pandemic?. *Transl Psychiatry* 6(3):e759. doi:10.1038/tp.2016.25.

Ley, R. E. et al. (2006). JI. Microbial ecology: human gut microbes associated with obesity. *Nature* 444(7122):1022–1023. doi:10.1038/4441022a.

Li, S. et al. (2010). NUTRIOSE dietary fiber supplementation improves insulin resistance and determinants of metabolic syndrome in overweight men: a double-blind, randomized, placebo-controlled study. *Appl Physiol Nutr Metab* 35(6):773–782. doi:10.1139/H10-074.

Li, Y. et al. (2017). Dietary patterns and depression risk: A meta-analysis. *Psychiatry Res* 253:373–82.

Lopes Sakamoto, F. et al. (2019). Psychotropic effects of L-theanine and its clinical properties: From the management of anxiety and stress to a potential use in schizophrenia. *Pharmacol Res* 147:104395. doi:10.1016/j.phrs.2019.104395. Epub 2019 Aug 11.

Luppino, F.S. et al. (2010). Overweight, obesity, and depression: a systematic review and meta-analysis of longitudinal studies. *Arch Gen Psychiatry* 67(3):220–229. doi:10.1001/archgenpsychiatry.2010.2.

Mahmood, A. et al. (2007). Zinc carnosine, a health food supplement that stabilises small bowel integrity and stimulates gut repair processes. *Gut* 56(2):168–75. doi:10.1136/gut.2006.099929. Epub 2006 Jun 15.

Mariat, D. et al. (2009). The Firmicutes/Bacteroidetes ratio of the human microbiota changes with age. *BMC Microbiol* 9:123. doi:10.1186/1471-2180-9-123.

McKean, J. et al. (2017). Probiotics and Subclinical Psychological Symptoms in Healthy Participants: A Systematic Review and Meta-Analysis. *J Altern Complement Med* 23(4):249–258. doi:10.1089/acm.2016.0023.

Messaoudi, M. et al. (2011). Assessment of psychotropic-like properties of a probiotic formulation (Lactobacillus helveticus R0052 and Bifidobacterium longum R0175) in rats and human subjects. *Br J Nutr* 105(5):755–64. doi:10.1017/S0007114510004319. Epub 2010 Oct 26.

Messaoudi, M. et al. (2011). Beneficial psychological effects of a probiotic formulation (Lactobacillus helveticus R0052 and Bifidobacterium longum R0175) in healthy human volunteers. *Gut Microbes* 2(4):256–261. doi:10.4161/gmic.2.4.16108.

Morris, M. C. et al. (2003). Dietary fats and the risk of incident Alzheimer disease. *Arch Neurol* 60(2):194–200.

Mudgil, D. et al. (2018). Partially hydrolyzed guar gum as a potential prebiotic source. *Int J Biol Macromol* 112:207–210. doi:10.1016/j.ijbiomac.2018.01.164.

Mulugeta, A. et al. (2018). Obesity and depressive symptoms in mid-life: a population-based cohort study. *BMC Psychiatry* 18(1):297. doi:10.1186/s12888-018-1877-6.

Muscogiuri, G. et al. (2019). Gut microbiota: a new path to treat obesity. *Int J Obes Suppl* 9(1):10–19. doi:10.1038/s41367-019-0011-7.

Nanri, A. et al. (2013). Dietary patterns and suicide in Japanese adults: the Japan Public Health Center-based Prospective Study. *Br J Psychiatry* 203:422–7.

Ng, Q. X. et al. (2018). A meta-analysis of the use of probiotics to alleviate depressive symptoms. *J Affect Disord* 228:13–19. doi:10.1016/j.jad.2017.11.063.

Niv, E. et al. (2016). Randomized clinical study: Partially hydrolyzed guar gum (PHGG) versus placebo in the treatment of patients with irritable bowel syndrome. *Nutr Metab* (Lond)13:10. doi:10.1186/s12986-016-0070-5.

Noto, H. et al. (2013). Low-carbohydrate diets and all-cause mortality: a systematic review and meta-analysis of observational studies. *PLoS One* 8(1): e55030.

Ohland, C.L. et al. (2013). Effects of Lactobacillus helveticus on murine behavior are dependent on diet and genotype and correlate with alterations in the gut microbiome. *Psychoneuroendocrinology* 38(9):1738–1747. doi:10.1016/j.psyneuen.2013.02.008.

Opie, R. et al. (2015). Assessing Healthy Diet Affordability in a Cohort with Major Depressive Disorder. *Journal of Public Health and Epidemiology* 7(5):159–69.

Osterberg, K.L. et al. (2015). Probiotic supplementation attenuates increases in body mass and fat mass during high-fat diet in healthy young adults. *Obesity* (Silver Spring) 23(12):2364–2370. doi:10.1002/oby.21230.

Park, E. et al. (2016). Effects of grape seed extract beverage on blood pressure and metabolic indices in individuals with pre-hypertension: a randomised, double-blinded, two-arm, parallel, placebo-controlled trial. *Br J Nutr* 115(2):226–38. doi:10.1017/S0007114515004328. Epub 2015 Nov 16.

Parletta, N. et al. (2017). A Mediterranean-style dietary intervention supplemented with fish oil improves diet quality and mental health in people with depression: A randomized controlled trial (HELFIMED). *Nutr Neurosci* 1–14.

Parnell, J. A. and R. A. Reimer. (2009). Weight loss during oligofructose supplementation is associated with decreased ghrelin and increased peptide YY in overweight and obese adults. *Am J Clin Nutr* 89(6):1751–1759. doi:10.3945/ajcn.2009.27465.

Pasco, J. A. et al. (2010). Association of high-sensitivity C-reactive protein with de novo major depression. *Br J Psychiatry* 197:372–7.

Peng, H. H. et al. (2019). Probiotic treatment restores normal developmental trajectories of fear memory retention in maternally separated infant rats. *Neuropharmacology* 153:53–62. doi:10.1016/j.neuropharm.2019.04.026. Epub 2019 Apr 26.

Pistell, P. J. et al. (2010). Cognitive impairment following high fat diet consumption is associated with brain inflammation. *J Neuroimmunol* 219(1–2):25–32.

Pittaway, J. K. et al. (2006). Dietary supplementation with chickpeas for at least 5 weeks results in small but significant reductions in serum total and low-density lipoprotein cholesterols in adult women and men. *Ann Nutr Metab* 50(6):512–8. doi:10.1159/000098143. Epub 2006 Dec 21.

Pittaway, J. K. et al. (2008). Chickpeas may influence fatty acid and fiber intake in an ad libitum diet, leading to small improvements in serum lipid profile and glycemic control. *J Am Diet Assoc* 108(6):1009–13. doi:10.1016/j.jada.2008.03.009.

Psaltopoulou, T. et al. (2013). Mediterranean diet, stroke, cognitive impairment, and depression: A meta-analysis. *Annals of Neurology* 74(4):580–91.

Rana, S. and S. Bhushan. (2016). Apple phenolics as nutraceuticals: assessment, analysis and application. *J Food Sci Technol* 53(4):1727–38. doi:10.1007/s13197-015-2093-8. Epub 2015 Nov 23.

Reichelt, A. C. and M. M. Rank (2017). The impact of junk foods on the adolescent brain. *Birth Defects Res* 109(20):1649–58.

Reid, S. N. S. et al. (2018). The Effects of Fermented Laminaria japonica on Short-Term Working Memory and Physical Fitness in the Elderly. *Evid Based Complement Alternat Med* 2018:8109621. doi:10.1155/2018/8109621.

Roman, B. E. et al. (2013). Short-term supplementation with active hexose correlated compound improves the antibody response to influenza B vaccine. *Nutr Res* 33(1):12–7. doi: 10.1016/j.nutres.2012.11.001. Epub 2012 Dec 4.

Romijn, A. R. et al. (2017). A double-blind, randomized, placebo-controlled trial of Lactobacillus helveticus and Bifidobacterium longum for the symptoms of depression. *Aust N Z J Psychiatry* 51(8):810–821. doi:10.1177/0004867416686694. Epub 2017 Jan 10.

Roshanravan, N. et al. (2017). Effect of Butyrate and Inulin Supplementation on Glycemic Status, Lipid Profile and Glucagon-Like Peptide 1 Level in Patients with Type 2 Diabetes: A Randomized Double-Blind, Placebo-Controlled Trial. *Horm Metab Res* 49(11):886–891. doi:10.1055/s-0043-119089. Epub 2017 Sep 29.

Rossi, V. and G. Pourtois. (2012). Transient state-dependent fluctuations in anxiety measured using STAI, POMS, PANAS or VAS: a comparative review. *Anxiety Stress Coping* 25(6):603–645. doi:10.1080/10615806.2011.582948.

Sanchez, M. et al. (2014). Effect of Lactobacillus rhamnosus CGMCC1.3724 supplementation on weight loss and maintenance in obese men and women. *Br J Nutr* 111(8):1507–1519. doi:10.1017/S0007114513003875.

Sanchez, M. et al. (2017). Effects of a Diet-Based Weight-Reducing Program with Probiotic Supplementation on Satiety Efficiency, Eating Behaviour Traits, and Psychosocial Behaviours in Obese Individuals. *Nutrients* 9(3):284. doi:10.3390/nu9030284.

Sanchez-Villegas, A. et al. (2009). Association of the Mediterranean dietary pattern with the incidence of depression: The Seguimiento Universidad de Navarra/ University of Navarra follow-up (SUN) cohort. *Archives of General Psychiatry* 66(10):1090–8.

Sanchez-Villegas, A. et al. (2013). Mediterranean dietary pattern and depression: the PREDIMED randomized trial. *BMC Med* 11:208.

Schachter, J. et al. (2018). Effects of obesity on depression: A role for inflammation and the gut microbiota. *Brain Behav Immun* 69:1–8. doi:10.1016/j.bbi.2017.08.026.

Schmidt, K. et al. (2015). Prebiotic intake reduces the waking cortisol response and alters emotional bias in healthy volunteers. *Psychopharmacology* (Berl) 232(10):1793–801. doi:10.1007/s00213-014-3810-0. Epub 2014 Dec 3.

Schwingshackl, L. and G. Hoffmann (2014). Mediterranean dietary pattern, inflammation and endothelial function: a systematic review and meta-analysis of intervention trials. *Nutr Metab Cardiovasc Dis* 24(9):929–39.

Siddarth, P. et al. (2020). Randomized placebo-controlled study of the memory effects of pomegranate juice in middle-aged and older adults. *Am J Clin Nutr* 111(1):170-177. doi: 10.1093/ajcn/nqz241.

Sivamaruthi, B. S. et al. (2019). Review on Role of Microbiome in Obesity and Antiobesity Properties of Probiotic Supplements. *Biomed Res Int* 2019:3291367. doi:10.1155/2019/3291367.

Smith, K. A. et al. (2000). Impaired regulation of brain serotonin function during dieting in women recovered from depression. *Br J Psychiatry* 176:72–75. doi:10.1192/bjp.176.1.72.

Spierings, E. L. et al. (2007). A Phase I study of the safety of the nutritional supplement, active hexose correlated compound, AHCC, in healthy volunteers. *J Nutr Sci Vitaminol* (Tokyo) 53(6):536–9. doi:10.3177/jnsv.53.536.

Stenman, L. K. et al. (2016). Probiotic With or Without Fiber Controls Body Fat Mass, Associated With Serum Zonulin, in Overweight and Obese Adults-Randomized Controlled Trial. *EBioMedicine* 190–200. doi:10.1016/j.ebiom.2016.10.036. Epub 2016 Oct 26.

Suez, J. et al. (2014). Artificial sweeteners induce glucose intolerance by altering the gut microbiota. *Nature* 514(7521):181–6.

Takanari, J. et al. (2016). Effect of Enzyme-Treated Asparagus Extract (ETAS) on Psychological Stress in Healthy Individuals. *J Nutr Sci Vitaminol* (Tokyo) 62(3):198–205. doi:10.3177/jnsv.62.198.

Talbott, S. and J. Talbott. (2009). Effect of BETA 1, 3/1, 6 GLUCAN on Upper Respiratory Tract Infection Symptoms and Mood State in Marathon Athletes. *J Sports Sci Med* 1;8(4):509–15.

Talbott, S. M. and J. A. Talbott. (2012). Baker's yeast beta-glucan supplement reduces upper respiratory symptoms and improves mood state in stressed women. *J Am Coll Nutr* 31(4):295–300. doi: 10.1080/07315724.2012.10720441.

Terakawa, N. et al. (2008). Immunological effect of active hexose correlated compound (AHCC) in healthy volunteers: a double-blind, placebo-controlled trial. *Nutr Cancer* 60(5):643–51.doi:10.1080/01635580801993280.

Terauchi, M. et al. (2014). Effects of grape seed proanthocyanidin extract on menopausal symptoms, body composition, and cardiovascular parameters in middle-aged women: a randomized, double-blind, placebo-controlled pilot study. *Menopause* 21(9):990–6. doi:10.1097/GME.0000000000000200.

Trošt, K. et al. (2018). Host: Microbiome co-metabolic processing of dietary polyphenols - An acute, single blinded, cross-over study with different doses of apple polyphenols in healthy subjects. *Food Res Int* 112:108–128. doi:10.1016/j.foodres.2018.06.016. Epub 2018 Jun 8.

Turnbaugh, P. J. et al. (2006). An obesity-associated gut microbiome with increased capacity for energy harvest. *Nature* 444(7122):1027–1031. doi:10.1038/nature05414.

Unno, K. et al. (2020). Theanine, the Main Amino Acid in Tea, Prevents Stress-Induced Brain Atrophy by Modifying Early Stress Responses. *Nutrients* 12(1):E174. doi:10.3390/nu12010174.

Valussi, M. (2012). Functional foods with digestion-enhancing properties. *Int J Food Sci Nutr* 63 Suppl 1:82–9. doi:10.3109/09637486.2011.627841. Epub 2011 Oct 19.

van der Beek, C. M. et al. (2018). The prebiotic inulin improves substrate metabolism and promotes short-chain fatty acid production in overweight to obese men. *Metabolism* 87:25–35. doi:10.1016/j.metabol.2018.06.009. Epub 2018 Jun 25.

Viveros, A. et al. (2011). Effects of dietary polyphenol-rich grape products on intestinal microflora and gut morphology in broiler chicks. *Poult Sci* 90(3):566–78. doi:10.3382/ps.2010-00889.

Walsh, A. M. et al. (2012). Effects of supplementing dietary laminarin and fucoidan on intestinal morphology and the immune gene expression in the weaned pig. *J Anim Sci* 90 Suppl 4:284-6. doi:10.2527/jas.53949.

World Health Organization (WHO) website (https://www.who.int/en/news-room/fact-sheets/detail/obesity-and-overweight; https://www.who.int/mental_health/management/depression/en/)—accessed December 1, 2019.

Wright, C. M. et al. (2019). Effect of a Fucoidan Extract on Insulin Resistance and Cardiometabolic Markers in Obese, Nondiabetic Subjects: A Randomized, Controlled Trial. *J Altern Complement Med* 25(3):346-352. doi:10.1089/acm.2018.0189. Epub 2018 Oct 12. PMID: 30312135.

Yang, X. D. et al. (2018). Effects of prebiotic galacto-oligosaccharide on postoperative cognitive dysfunction and neuroinflammation through targeting of the gut-brain axis. *BMC Anesthesiol* 18(1):177. doi:10.1186/s12871-018-0642-1.

Yasukawa, Z. et al. (2019). Effect of Repeated Consumption of Partially Hydrolyzed Guar Gum on Fecal Characteristics and Gut Microbiota: A Randomized, Double-Blind, Placebo-Controlled, and Parallel-Group Clinical Trial. *Nutrients* 11(9):2170. doi:10.3390/nu11092170.

Zembron-Lacny, A. et al. (2013). Effect of shiitake (Lentinus edodes) extract on antioxidant and inflammatory response to prolonged eccentric exercise. *J Physiol Pharmacol* 64(2):249–54.

INDEX

ABOUT THE AUTHOR

Dr. Shawn Talbott received dual Bachelor's degrees in Sports Medicine (B.S.) and Fitness Management (B.A.) from Marietta College, his Master's degree (M.S.) in Exercise Science from the University of Massachusetts, and his Ph.D. in Nutritional Biochemistry from Rutgers University. His research is primarily focused on natural products (dietary supplements, herbal medicine, and functional foods) to support psychological vigor (physical energy, mental acuity, and emotional well-being) as well as metabolism, weight loss, stress resilience, sports nutrition, and human performance.

Dr. Talbott is also a Diplomate of the International Olympic Committee's (IOC) Sports Nutrition program, and has studied Entrepreneurship at the Massachusetts Institute of Technology (MIT), including the Entrepreneurial Masters Program (EMP), the Entrepreneurship Development Program (EDP), and the Advanced Certificate for Executives (ACE) in Management, Innovation, and Technology.

He has served as a nutrition educator for elite-level athletes in a variety of sports:

➤ Professional triathletes (including Ironman podiums)

➤ Members of the Utah Jazz (NBA basketball)

➤ United States Ski & Snowboard Association during the 2002 Winter Olympics

➤ Performance Enhancement Team (PET) for the U.S. Track & Field Association

➤ The United States Olympic Training Center (Chula Vista, CA)

➤ Members of Real Salt Lake (Major League Soccer)

➤ As an athlete himself, Shawn is the 2014 "World's Fittest CEO" and has competed at the national and international level in:

➤ Rowing (as part of the U.S. National Team Development Program)

➤ Cycling (at the Lake Placid Olympic Training Center Development Program)

➤ Triathlon (holding a professional license for 2 years and completing over 100 marathons, ultra-marathons, and triathlons, including 18 at the Ironman distance)

He is a Fellow of the American College of Nutrition (ACN), the American College of Sports Medicine (ACSM), and the American Institute of Stress (AIS).

As a product developer, Dr. Talbott has created and researched some of the leading nutritional products on the market, generating over $1 billion in combined sales.

Dr. Talbott's recent educational projects include two academic textbooks, an award-winning documentary film, and several best-selling books that have been translated into multiple languages. His work to educate people about nutrition and health has been featured on The Dr. Oz Show, the TED stage, and the White House.

He lives with his family in Utah and Massachusetts.